GENDER-AFFIRMING SURGERIES

Planning through Post-op for Transgender and Gender-Nonconforming Adults

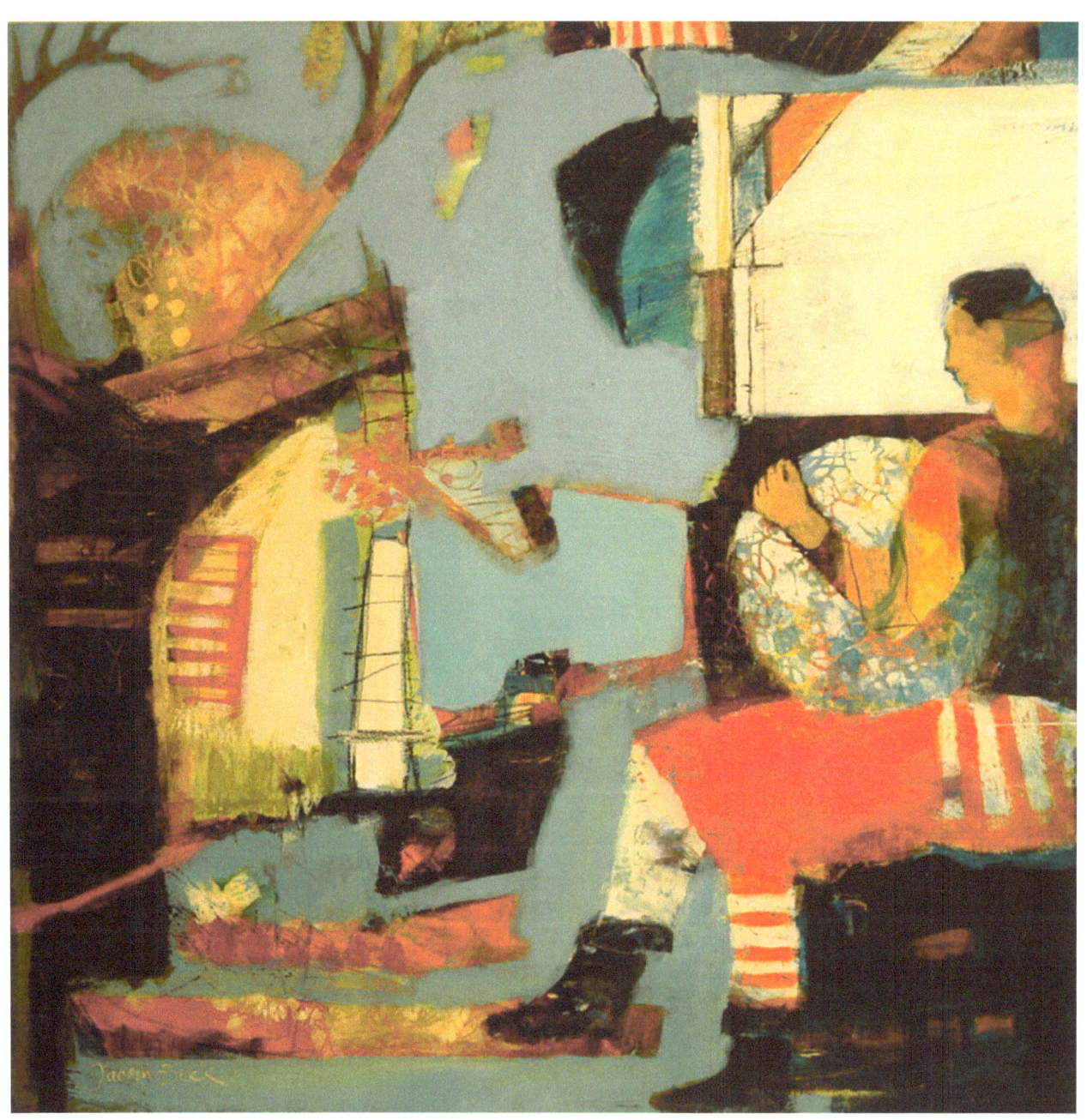

Holding the World

GENDER-AFFIRMING SURGERIES

Planning through Post-op for Transgender and Gender-Nonconforming Adults

Linda Gromko, MD

A NOTE ABOUT THIS BOOK

This book contains sections relating to surgery and post-op care that appear in
A Practical Reference for Transgender and Gender-Nonconforming Adults,
a comprehensive guide to healthcare and navigating daily life
for the transgender and gender-nonconforming adult.

OTHER BOOKS BY LINDA GROMKO, MD

A Practical Reference for Transgender and Gender-Nonconforming Adults

Complications: A Doctor's Love Story

*Let Me Go When the Banter Stops:
A Doctor's Fight for the Love of Her Life*

*Arranging Your Life When Dialysis Comes Home:
The Underwear Factor*
by Linda Gromko, MD and Jane C. McClure

*Where's MY Book? A Guide for Transgender and Gender Non-Conforming Youth,
Their Parents, & Everyone Else*

Bainbridge Books, Seattle, Washington
Copyright © 2022 Linda Gromko, MD

Cover image by Jacqui Beck

Print edition ISBN: 978-0-9825143-6-8
eBook edition ISBN: 978-0-9825143-3-7
Library of Congress Control Number: 2022911250

MEDICAL DISCLAIMER
This book contains general information about gender dysphoria and related medical and surgical topics. It discusses depression, suicidality, sexuality, sexually transmitted infections, and a range of other health-related topics.

This book should not, however, be relied upon to diagnose or treat any illness, condition, or disease—or to manage any postoperative complications. This is what your healthcare providers are for! Consult your healthcare practitioner before beginning any new diet or exercise program. Certainly, take this book to your healthcare provider with your questions about anything in this book. I heartily encourage you not to purchase medications online without the assistance of your healthcare provider.

The author and contributors disclaim any liability or responsibility for injury or damage to persons or property incurred, directly or indirectly, from application of any of the contents of this book. It is the reader's responsibility to know and follow the recommendations of their healthcare providers who have specific knowledge of the reader's circumstances.

DEDICATION

**This book is gratefully dedicated to my friend, David,
who has taught me important lessons about gender and life.**

David carved out a unique life against steep odds. He transitioned in young adulthood at a time when very few people managed that. He became an accomplished scientist. He married his soulmate Ann, loving her throughout their life together and after her death. David nurtured his golden retriever "soul dog" Sam and later a rambunctious puppy named "M."

When I met him, David was in his early seventies, moving through his stealth life with stubbornness and courage. He actively pursued personal growth, reading extensively and conquering the goblins of childhood. His world expanded with improving health, regular swimming, and new and old friendships alike.

David began attending trans support meetings at Ingersoll Gender Center. He became a champion of the youth book I wrote, *Where's MY Book? A Guide for Transgender and Gender Non-Conforming Youth, Their Parents, & Everyone Else*, donating copies for fundraising raffles and recommending it to parents of trans youth.

In December 2019, David suffered an unthinkable accident. At home alone with M, David fell—driving his hard head nearly through a plasterboard wall. He landed on his face and knees, his neck bent. He couldn't move at all. He couldn't have summoned anyone even if he had had his phone. Four days after the accident, a swimming buddy (Judy) thought it odd that David hadn't come to the pool. It was she who initiated the police welfare check that saved David's life. The police found an immobile David and his loudly barking M. The medics transferred David to the hospital.

David had become a high quadriplegic in that split-second horror. With blood clots in his legs and his lungs, he clearly should have died. But he didn't die.

Suddenly, "stealth" in any fashion was impossible and no longer protective of anything. Literally everything was exposed. But minute to minute, David landed on metaphorical feet, forging on with that stubborn head and sincere heart. I have never seen anyone quite as durable as David.

I know David likes the idea of the adult trans book. So, to him, and in honor of all who have survived against steep odds, I dedicate this effort.

Happy Birthday, my friend.

David died on March 6, 2021—15 months after his paralyzing fall. I arrived a few minutes after he died, helped the caregivers bathe him, and stood witness as the mortuary person zipped him into the blanket body bag. It was important to me that David's body was treated respectfully.

I had had my weekly conversation with David just two afternoons before. We talked about his medications, we talked about pain, and we talked about his phlegm. But David had had a dream, and he was eager to share it with me. Working to push out his breaths and speaking with a gravelly voice, he told me the dream.

"I was in the midst of being born. My head was out, and I could see light and color—it was beautiful. And I really got it what love is. Love is total trust.

"It felt like I knew God and God is trust. I was surrounded by love—everyone I have ever known; people I've read about, like Gandhi and Martin Luther King. And my wife Ann. It was wonderful to see her again. She was the same as before; she was 40.

"The ultimate lesson is that God is love and God is total trust. This has changed my life already. I am more comfortable, not afraid of dying—this revelation took away the fear. I want to live and live this [world view] many more days. I want to tell the people I trust. I told my caregivers. It all makes sense. This gift is why I'm alive."

The dream had changed David, washing away his PTSD, washing away his fears. I often wondered why David had lived through his horrific accident, why he lived through the custom karmic hell of total dependency. And now, I knew.

Rest in peace, David.

— Linda Gromko, MD

TABLE OF CONTENTS

Dedication v
Preface xii
Introduction xxi

CHAPTER 1 | Planning for Your Surgery 1
   Waiting for Your Gender-Affirming Surgery 1
   The Critical 1 to 2 Years before Surgery 1
   Your Personal Goals 2
      What Do You Hope Your Surgery Will Accomplish? 2
      How Realistic Are Your Hopes and Expectations? 2
      If You Are Envisioning Multiple Surgeries, Where Will You Start? 2
      Are Your Goals Reachable by Surgery? 3
      Do the Collective Benefits of Surgery Outweigh the Risks for You? 3
   Optimizing Your Personal Health before Surgery 3
      Get a Thorough Medical Evaluation 3
      Laboratory Tests for a General Evaluation 4
      Other Medical Conditions to Be Evaluated before Surgery 4
   Modify Any Personal Health Habits That May Impact Your Surgical Risks 7
      Stop Smoking Now If You Smoke (Tobacco, Marijuana, Hookahs) or Use Tobacco Products 7
      Help with Quitting Smoking 8
      Manage Your Weight 9
         Help with Weight Loss 9
      Address Your Alcohol Intake 11
      Know Your STI (STD) Status 11
      Allow at Least a Year for Hair Removal If Your Surgeon Requires Hair Removal for Genital Surgery 11
      Optimize Your Physical Fitness 12
      Check Your Immunization Status 12
   Paying for Your Surgery 12
      Find a Trans-Advocacy Legal Organization to Help You Understand Your Insurance 13
      Surgery Itself Is Only *One* Expense 13
      Other Ways to Help Cover Surgical and Nonsurgical Costs (Besides Insurance) 14
   Choosing Your Surgeon 16
      Getting Your Presurgery Letters 19
      Practical Pointers to Help You Get Your Letters 19
   The Critical 6 Weeks Prior to Surgery 20
      Confirm Logistical Arrangements with Your Surgeon's Office 20
      Confirm Medical Arrangements with Your Surgeon's Office 21
      Confirm Your Travel Arrangements 23
      Confirm Work Arrangements 23
      Being Discreet 24
      Other Preoperative Considerations 25
      Helping Others Help You 26
      Shopping Lists for Surgery 27

CHAPTER 2 | Feminizing Surgeries 29
   Disclaimer 29
   Facial Feminization Surgery 30

- FFS Is a Collection of Surgeries...33
- Vocal Feminization Surgery and ET Tubes...36
- Breast Enlargement (Augmentation Mammoplasty)...36
  - The Rice Test: Determining Breast Size and Breast Implant Size...38
  - Possible Complications Associated with Breast Implants...39
  - Breast Implant-Associated Anaplastic Large-Cell Lymphoma (BIA-ALCL)...41
- Body Contouring...41
  - Nonsurgical Body Contouring...41
  - Surgical Body Contouring...41
  - Risks of Tumescent Liposuction...42
  - Doing the Math: Is an Aesthetic Procedure Worth It?...43
  - More Body Contouring: Lifting and Filling...43
    - Be an Informed Consumer...44
    - An Important Warning about Liquid Silicone Injections...44
- Feminizing Genital Surgeries...44
  - Orchiectomy...44
  - Vaginoplasty...45
  - Learning about the Feminizing Genital Surgeries...48
  - Animation Videos of Vaginoplasty...48
  - One-Stage Penile Inversion Vaginoplasty...49
  - What Happens to the Prostate?...53
  - Two-Stage Vaginoplasty (Penile Inversion Vaginoplasty Plus Labiaplasty Done Later)...53
  - The Limited-Depth or Zero-Depth Vagina...54
  - Vaginoplasty with Limited Graft Tissue...54
  - The Peritoneal Pull-Through Vaginoplasty...55
    - Perineum versus Peritoneum: Big Difference!...55
  - Vaginoplasty Using the Sigmoid Colon (Rectosigmoid Vaginoplasty)...57
  - Vaginoplasty Using the Right (Ascending) Colon: aka Right Colo-Vaginoplasty...58
    - Potential Advantages of the Right-Colon Vaginoplasty...59
    - Potential Disadvantages...59
  - Dr. Alvaro H. Rodriguez Introduces Vaginoplasty Grafts from Tilapia...60

CHAPTER 3 | Masculinizing Surgeries...63
- Disclaimer...63
  - Facial Masculinization Surgery...63
    - FMS Is a Collection of Surgeries...65
  - Gender-Affirming Chest Reconstruction (Top Surgery)...66
    - Postsurgical Scars in Reduction Mammoplasty versus Top Surgery...66
    - Bidding the Girls—but Not My Personality—Goodbye...68
  - Hysterectomy and Bilateral Salpingo-Oophorectomy...69
  - Monsplasty...70
  - Laparoscopy and Robot-Assisted Surgeries...70
  - Learning about the Masculinizing Genital Surgeries...71
- Masculinizing Genital Surgeries...72
- Deciding on the Best Type of Masculinizing Genital Surgery for You...72
  - Answer the Following Questions about Your Own Goals...72
  - Deciding on a Type of Male Genital Surgery (Table)...73
  - Metoidioplasty (Also Known as "Meta")...74
    - Metoidioplasty with Urethral Extension (Also Called Urethral Lengthening)...74
    - Metoidioplasty and Scrotoplasty with or without Testicular Implants...75
  - Expectations for Metoidioplasty and Its Variations...75

Phalloplasty...76
　Some Important Surgical Definitions..76
　Skin Grafts and Flaps..76
　　Definition of a Graft..77
　　Definition of a Flap...77
　Phalloplasty Options...78
　　All Phalloplasties Require Several Steps...................................79
　　Radial Forearm Flap Phalloplasty (RFF).....................................79
　　　First Stage: Phallus Creation..79
　　　Second Stage: Urethral Lengthening and Scrotoplasty......................81
　　　Third Stage: Erectile Implant..82
　　Shower or Grower?..83
　　Anterior Lateral Thigh Flap Phalloplasty...................................84
　　The Delayed Pedicle(d) Flap Phalloplasty (Also Called a Local Flap Phalloplasty).........84
　A Surgeon's Advice...87
　Managing the Expectations of Phalloplasty....................................87
Nonbinary (or Less Binary) Genital Surgeries...................................88
　Penile Preservation Vaginoplasty with Peritoneal Pull-Through: Something New......88
　The Penis/Phallus-Preserving Vaginoplasty with Peritoneal Pull-Through.......88
　　The Penis/Phallus-Preserving Vaginoplasty with Full-Thickness Skin Graft...88
　Gender Nullification Surgery: "The Smoothie"................................89

CHAPTER 4 | In Case of Emergencies..91
Recognizing When You Are in Trouble: Emergency Warnings That Apply to All Surgeries......91
　Post and Keep Emergency Information on Your Phone...........................91
　When to Call 911..91
　What Happens If You Call 911 and It Turns Out to Be a False Alarm?..........93
　Other Urgent Situations You Might Encounter.................................93
　　You Are Suicidal..93
　　You Are Having Pain...93
　　You Have a Fever..94
　　You Are Having Nausea, Vomiting, and Diarrhea and Are Feeling Progressively Weaker......94
　　You Are Having Urinary Symptoms...94

CHAPTER 5 | Taking Care of Yourself after Surgery.............................97
What to Expect in the Hospital...97
　You Will Likely Follow the Standard Routine.................................97
　After Surgery, You Will Be Moved into the Recovery Room or the Postanesthesia Recovery Area......99
　When You Are Awake and Breathing without Assistance.........................99
General Postoperative Home Care Guidelines for *All* Surgeries................100
　It Can Take a Village: Your Team of Support................................100
　Planning the Length of Your Recovery Time..................................102
　Resting Effectively after Surgery..102
　Managing Postoperative Pain..104
　Postoperative Nutrition: Getting Enough Protein for Wound Healing..........106
　　Protein Content of Various Foods from Animal and Plant Sources (Table)...107
　　Drink Your Protein...108
　Getting Enough Fluid...108
　　Volume Depletion and Dehydration: Not the Same Thing....................108
　Caring for Your Wounds...110

Changing Your Dressings: The Very Basics 111
Gentle Attention to Your Mental Health 113
Are You Depressed? 114
Recognize That You Are at Risk 114

CHAPTER 6 | Specific Postoperative Circumstances Dealing with Specific Surgeries 117
Feminizing Surgeries 117
Facial Feminization Surgery: Post-Op Considerations 117
Here Are Some Pointers to Help You after Facial Feminization Surgery 117
Patience Is Critical! 118
Breast Augmentation Surgery 119
Orchiectomy 119
Vaginoplasty 119
Does My Vagina Look Normal? 119
Dilation Is Critical 120
Follow Your Surgeon's Dilation Instructions Precisely 121
Helpful Pointers for Dilation after Vaginoplasty 121
Dilation Q & A 122
Learning to Pee after Vaginoplasty 123
Watch for the Following UTI Warnings 123
Swelling in the Perineum 124
Constipation in the Postoperative Period 124
Common Worries 125
If Your Sutures Are Coming Out or the Incision Is Opening 125
If You Experience Vaginal Bleeding or See a Streak of Blood on Your Dilator 125
Peritoneal Pull-Through Vaginoplasty and Phallus-Preserving Peritoneal Pull-Through 125
Masculinizing Surgeries 125
Facial Masculinization Surgery 126
After Gender-Affirming Chest Reconstruction (Top Surgery) 126
After Hysterectomy and Bilateral Salpingo-Oophorectomy 127
After Monsplasty 128
After Vaginectomy 129
After Metoidioplasty 129
After Metoidioplasty with Urethral Extension (Lengthening) 129
After Scrotoplasty with Prosthetic Testes Placed 130
After Phalloplasty (Free Forearm Flap and Anterior Lateral Thigh Flap) 130
What Is a Wound VAC? 133
Urinary Leakage after Phalloplasty 133
After a Delayed Pedicle Flap Phalloplasty 133
Phallus Tattoos: A Game Changer 134
Quest House: A Post-Op Home for Transmasculine and Nonbinary Individuals Recovering
from Phalloplasty and Other Gender-Affirming Surgeries near San Francisco 135

Conclusion 141
List of Figures and Tables 142
Bibliography 143
Photo and Illustration Credits 145
Acknowledgments 146
Index 149
About the Author 156
About Artist Jacqui Beck 157

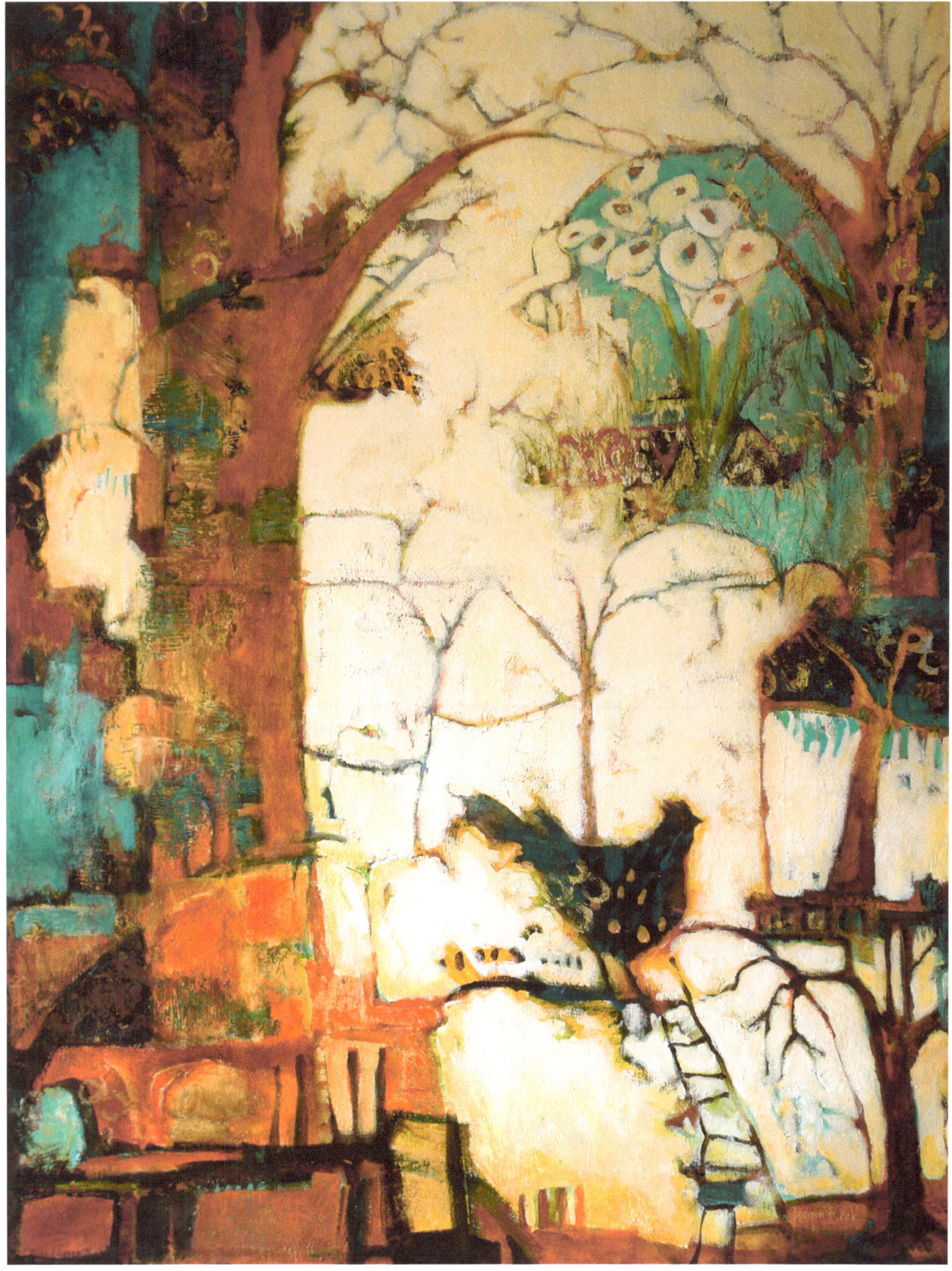

Tree House

PREFACE

A Practical Reference for Transgender Adults from an Elder Cisgender Medical Doctor

I've been involved in healthcare since I was a candy striper some 50 years ago. I graduated with a bachelor's in nursing from the University of Washington in 1973 and completed the University of Washington Family Nurse Practitioner Program in its infancy in 1975. It was during my years as a nurse practitioner and educator at Planned Parenthood that I identified a true calling to go to medical school. Not as an escape. I loved everything I did in nursing, but simply wanted to extend the depth and breadth of what I knew.

With a 2-year-old son in tow, I went back to school for the painful science prerequisites: a couple more years of chemistry, a couple of calculus courses, and a year each of physics and biology. My nursing background bought me no credit in the medical school entrance process. One advisor told me, "the kind of people who become nurses aren't the kind of people who become physicians!"

But when I started as a first-year University of Washington medical student in 1980, I realized instantly that my nursing background brought me solid advantages. For one thing, I was fluent in *speaking and writing medicine*—and its many abbreviations and expressions. Moreover, I knew how medical tasks got done, and I knew how the medical hierarchy operated.

Clinically, I had performed some 3,000 pelvic exams (and examined twice as many breasts) as a nurse practitioner at Planned Parenthood. I could confirm the duration of pregnancies with reasonable accuracy and could manage contraceptive options and treat sexually transmitted infections by rote.

Most of all, however, I recognized that my nursing background gave me the capacity to walk into any patient room at any time with something *to offer—even if that was purely my ability to interpret the language of medicine.*

After finishing medical school in 1984, I selected the University of Washington Family Practice Residency Program because I truly enjoyed all my clinical rotations in medical school. While I was drawn to obstetrics and women's healthcare, I didn't want to exclude men or children from my practice. I sought out additional experiences in psychiatry and surgery, gaining hours of extra experience in these areas.

The decision to go into family medicine wasn't a given, even at the University of Washington, which is widely known as one of the best primary care schools in the nation. When I was in medical school and expressed an interest in primary care, I remember a senior surgeon commenting, "Family practice—you'll be able to do a lot of things—*poorly.*"

But I knew then—and have confirmed time and time again—that there is a critical need for first-rate generalists. Our training and experience *do* stress breadth over depth, so we primary care providers are the ones who naturally scan and see the larger picture, much as the emergency room physician does. We may be the ones who save your medical neck because we haven't forgotten to look at all the medications or treatments in your medical scenario. We may be the ones who *interpret* diagnoses and treatments on behalf of some of our specialist colleagues. And when longevity of care is involved, we are the ones who can celebrate your personal victories and ache with you in your losses because we've been right there *with* you over the years.

Besides, when you're on an airplane and a medical crisis unfolds, does the flight attendant ask if there's an ophthalmologist (eye specialist) on the plane? For my money, I hope there's a family medicine or internal medicine provider or an emergency room doctor—someone with the "scanning" skills to size up the total picture quickly and move on to a logical plan.

Good healthcare requires both *general* and *specialty care*. Neither is done in a vacuum, and neither is more important than the other. What is important is knowing what is needed for a particular patient at a particular time.

After completing my family practice residency at the University of Washington, I worked for a couple of years as an emergency room physician, and as a "moonlighter" in a clinic that defended women's reproductive freedoms. These experiences enhanced my knowledge base and procedural skills—and confirmed my gut sense that I was cut out to work for myself (perhaps not unemployable but destined to be my own boss).

I opened my sturdy little family practice in 1989, located on the foot of Seattle's Queen Anne Hill, the neighborhood where I went to high school in the 1960s. We are still located there today, 30 years later.

From experience, I now understand why doctors may *not* wish to open their own independent practices. A small medical practice is a complicated little business: gritty and rugged and fraught with insurance struggles. There's a bit of financial skydiving required with no safety nets or subsidies to protect a small independent clinic. And, as in any small business, the owner is paid last—*after* we make the staff payroll. Intent on "doing the right thing," our practice covered the staff's medical and dental insurance from day one, and the practice payroll most certainly went on my personal Visa card from time to time.

But with several superb nurse practitioners and a seasoned and loyal staff, I can attest that opening an independent family medicine practice was the perfect choice *for me*. This style of practice suited *my* temperament. It satisfied my requirement to respond urgently to patient needs without having to okay reasonable policies with anyone other than myself and my colleagues, and perhaps my malpractice insurance carrier. The "higher power" I answered to was the standard of excellent medical care. My style of practice honored a clear commitment to doing what was right for each patient at a given time. And the small size of our practice made us nimble: able to recognize problems and find practical solutions by the close of the business day.

Over the years, I have learned that family practice is messy. Humans are complicated. Responding to humans' needs and doing our level best to help them through crises takes time. We have found consistently that no single protocol fits all people. *Human time and consideration will always be the currency of exchange in good medicine.*

I have noticed that the patients who seek out care in *our* practice are sincere, contributory individuals who truly aim to make the world a better place. Rather than seeing themselves as victims of circumstance, *our* patients tend to roll up their sleeves and work on their problems. And my staff and I ride right alongside them whether the issue is a problem pregnancy, a learning variance, a career mismatch, a relationship struggle, mental illness, alcohol dependency, aging parents, or the desire to navigate the end of life with as much control as a human can have.

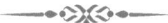

One day in 1998, a caller asked our receptionist, "Does Dr. Gromko treat transgender women?"

When the receptionist asked me the caller's question, I replied, "Not yet."

But I asked the receptionist to explain to the client that I was an absolute beginner in the field, and that I would be learning right along with her, and that I was likely to be learning *from* her. The caller said she was okay with all of that; very few Seattle doctors provided care for transgender clients. While I wouldn't choose to require a patient to become my teacher, it seems valid that we *always* learn from our patients. Truly, we don't stop learning until we stop listening.

As I write this, I recall that there *had* been another transgender woman who had asked if I would take her on as a patient. And I had said "no." After all, I had no training in transgender medicine in either my nursing or my medical education. At the time, it seemed medically appropriate—even responsible—to decline.

But by the time the second woman asked, perhaps only months later, it occurred to me that *my* comfort level was going to have to take second place. Here were real patients who needed care that I could learn to provide, even if it meant structuring my own learning.

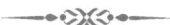

Setting out to learn about transgender medicine, I contacted the three physicians I knew who might know something, *anything*, about it. I read the WPATH Standards of Care. (The World Professional Association for Transgender Health, formerly the Harry Benjamin Society, has grown to be *the* international organization that serves as a clearinghouse and educational resource for clinicians.)

Locally, I contacted Marsha Botzer, the founder of Seattle's Ingersoll Gender Center. Marsha started Ingersoll in 1979 as a self-help organization that facilitated support groups and provided participants the limited information available on where to seek therapy and medical care, and even less information on surgical care.

Marsha invited me to attend a Friday night Open Group to learn more about the transgender community. The groups typically start with an around-the-group check-in, followed by a second hour focusing on a specific issue of the group's choosing.

I went to one group and just kept going every Friday evening for several months. This became the true foundation of my transgender education.

In the group, I learned about "gatekeeping." At the time, transgender people were required to work with a therapist for a minimum of 3 months and obtain a letter in support of receiving hormone therapy. While I've always been an advocate of counseling for *everybody*, it seemed that the policy could create an adversarial relationship between therapists and clients and between clients and prescribers. I believe the policy may have sent some folks to the Internet to prescribe their own hormones, something I've seen occur less often as time has passed. Worst of all, gatekeeping seemed to imply that a client couldn't be trusted to know what was best for them.

In the groups, I learned the impact that "coming out as trans" had on relationships, particularly with spouses and children. When I joined the group in 1999, couples seemed to split apart, as if by default. It was agonizing. Over the years, this has seemed far less automatic; many people are realizing that *it's the person, not the gender identity* that counts. And many more people now seem to find that the financial realities and emotional costs of breaking up a long-term relationship are simply too high. Today, I see more couples redefining their partnerships, either expanding their own sexual identities or recharacterizing their relationships as platonic.

I learned about the day-to-day struggles of transitioning. One woman described her three painful facial electrolysis treatments per week. (Having undergone a few upper-lip electrolysis treatments in college myself, this alone would have sealed my understanding that transitioning was not "a phase.") I heard the heartbreak of casual insults and the anguish of poorly concealed slights in the workplace. I witnessed the financial hardships experienced by people even trying to get the required therapist's letter to begin hormone therapy, let alone pay for their hormones or surgeries. Such services were almost never covered back then, although they are increasingly covered now.

The most critical point I discovered in the group was that a person's gender identity is not elective. It is not a discretionary definition that a person chooses. Certainly, an individual may elect to enter into the process of gender transition. But I learned that *that* decision—that is, to transition or not—was often a life-or-death matter.

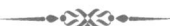

Armed with my embryonic awareness of the transgender community, I began to see more transgender clients. Word spread that there was a family doctor who had *some* information and was open to treating trans patients.

I remember the first trans male I treated. I called the University of Washington's Medcon service (a telephone consulting service for area providers) to get the little information they had, and I reviewed recommended testosterone dosing with a willing ally.

My client signed the consent form I had written (and reviewed with Ingersoll and my malpractice company). The clinic was so busy on that particular day that I had to meet my client in the clinic's baby room, which had a climbing ladder on the exam table and a floor-to-ceiling giraffe graphic in the corner. I apologized to the client, thinking he might have felt belittled by the ambiance of the infant room. But he just smiled and said,

"Well, it sort of *is* my birthday!"

From that moment on, I knew we'd be fine. Our intentions were evident, and our clientele was grateful.

In 2009, I was approached by Aidan Key, the founder of Gender Odyssey, an internationally known Seattle conference dealing with transgender issues. Aidan is also the founder of Gender Diversity, a support group network for transgender children and their parents.

It had become clear to Aidan that there was a need for providers who were willing and able to treat transgender adolescents with puberty blockers and cross-sex hormones. Aidan facilitated a trip for me and a local naturopathic physician, Christopher Bosted, ND, to travel with Aidan to Vancouver, British Columbia, to meet with Dan Metzger, MD, a Canadian endocrinologist who was an expert in the field. From Dan, I was able to learn important basic information and to confirm my understanding that many children were aware of gender asynchrony from toddlerhood.

From my practice, I had witnessed repeatedly the despair of trans women who had ached to forestall the onset of secondary sex characteristics like facial hair, height, stereotypically male facial features, and a deep voice. I could attest to the misery I witnessed in trans men wearing chest binders or having menstrual periods they hated. What a benefit it might be for some of my clients to reach their gender goals at an age where costly surgeries would not become necessary, where living a *lifetime* in their true gender was a possibility.

Since then, I have learned to insert the implantable histrelin puberty blockers into the arms of early-puberty kids, to give them the gift of "pausing" the puberty process. I typically also start cross-sex hormones in young adolescents, provided they and their parents are clear and well-informed.

In 2015, I published a book entitled *Where's MY Book? A Guide for Transgender and Gender Non-Conforming Youth, Their Parents, & Everyone Else*.

My reasons for writing the book were starkly clear to me.

> **Maybe it will become common for a teenager to say,**
> **"I've always been male, but I was born with female genitals."**

For one thing, a 17-year-old trans male in our practice died by suicide. He had orchestrated his death using helium suffocation; it was not an impulsive act. In his suicide note, the young man had written that one of his greatest concerns was that he would be misgendered after death! We never saw the suicide coming, and it broke my heart. (We know that nearly half of all transgender individuals have made a suicide attempt.)[1]

The second reason was that the puberty class presented at Seattle's Children's Hospital featured the popular book *Will Puberty Last My Whole Life?* by Julie Metzger, RN, MN, and Robert Lehman, MD. It was written directly from questions that arose from the actual puberty classes, so it was reality-based. But one

---

[1] Statistics for adolescent suicide attempts from 2015 data: "Nearly 14% of adolescents reported a previous suicide attempt; disparities by gender identity in suicide attempts were found. Female to male adolescents reported the highest rate of attempted suicide (50.8%), followed by adolescents who identified as not exclusively male or female (41.8%), male to female adolescents (29.9%), questioning adolescents (27.9%), female adolescents (17.6%), and male adolescents (9.8%)." Russell B. Toomey, Amy K. Syvertsen, and Maura Shramko, "Transgender Adolescent Suicide Behavior," *Pediatrics* 142, no. 4 (October 2018): 1, https://doi.org/10.1542/peds.2017-4218.
   Statistics for adult suicide attempts from 2015 data: "In a national study, 40% of transgender adults reported having made a suicide attempt. 92% of these individuals reported having attempted suicide before the age of 25." Sandy E. James et al., *The Report of the 2015 U.S. Transgender Survey* (Washington, DC: National Center for Transgender Equality, 2016), 24, https://transequality.org/sites/default/files/docs/usts/USTS-Full-Report-Dec17.pdf. Please also see https://www.thetrevorproject.org/resources/guide/preventing-suicide/.
   An analysis of the National Transgender Discrimination Survey (NTDS) from 2008 cites the following statistics: "Suicide attempts among trans men (46%) and trans women (42%) were slightly higher than the full sample (41%)...the prevalence of suicide attempts is elevated among those who disclose to everyone that they are transgender or gender-nonconforming (50%)." Jody L. Herman, Ann P. Haas, and Philip L. Rodgers, *Suicide Attempts among Transgender and Gender Non-Conforming Adults* (Los Angeles: The Williams Institute, UCLA, 2014), 2, https://escholarship.org/uc/item/8xg8061f.

half of the book was rimmed in blue for boys and the other half in raspberry pink for girls. There was little information on sexual orientation and nothing at all on gender diversity. (In fairness, this has changed some with the latest edition.)

I knew from experience that the kids I treated had been all over the Internet by the time they consulted me about gender dysphoria; they needed something more suited for them. So, *Where's MY Book? A Guide for Transgender and Gender Non-Conforming Youth, Their Parents, & Everyone Else* was born. I rated the book "R" for "Realistic."

I loved the book because it was conversational in tone and resonated with the gentle but realistic information we shared with our own patients. The book was beautifully sprinkled with the whimsical paintings of Seattle artist Jacqui Beck, who created her collection "Gender Personal" when her own child transitioned. I also appreciated the many contributions from staff, colleagues, and patients as they shared stories and practical tips to make the book more useful. Factual information on hormones, presentation, and surgery collided with the "Surviving and Thriving" chapters to create a work that has served families across the country, one Amazon purchase at a time.

The book was recognized with several awards in 2016: the ASSECT (American Association of Sexuality Educators, Counselors, and Therapists) Book of the Year; two Benjamin Franklin Silver Medals from the Independent Book Publishers Association in the categories of LGBT and Teen Nonfiction; a Gold Medal in the Global eBook competition in the category of LGBT Nonfiction; and First Place in the Health Category of the Eric Hoffer Book Award.

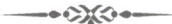

Through the years of the practice, we saw more and more trans women and trans men who were having gender-reassignment surgeries, both pre- and postoperatively.

One of the requisites for the surgical creation of a vagina, or vaginoplasty—at least with most surgeons—is the removal of genital hair by electrolysis or laser. The consequence of not having adequate hair removal before surgery is hair in the vagina after vaginoplasty, or medically worse, hair in the urethra after phalloplasty (the surgical creation of a penis).

One day in about 2013, I was prescribing EMLA cream (a topical numbing medicine) and a narcotic pain reliever for one of my patients to address pain during electrolysis.

In a light-bulb moment, I thought, *We could do this. And not only could we do this, we could do electrolysis and laser in-house with better anesthetic options.*

It was then that I personally took electrolysis training, as required by my malpractice insurance carrier. My partner-in-crime was one of our receptionists, Lauren Christophersen, who also trained. Lauren, it turned out, was an electrolysis savant—she was amazingly skilled right from the start.

Our practice bought two electrolysis machines. We also bought a Vectus laser that was designed exclusively for hair removal.

Then we addressed the issue of pain management. I desperately wanted hair removal in my clinic *not* to represent "yet another punishment for being transgender." My cosmetic surgery colleague, Tony Mangubat,

MD, gave me the recipe for an effective prescription-strength topical medication called "BLT" (benzocaine, lidocaine, tetracaine) that could be used before painful treatments.

While at a WPATH conference in Bangkok in 2014, I spoke with surgeon Toby Meltzer. Toby showed me how to perform a spermatic cord block on a napkin during a dinner cruise. We've modified our technique over the years to do mostly scrotal field blocks, but it was a tremendous start. We have some clients who sleep through their electrolysis treatments.

Then, in Seattle, I asked the dentist upstairs in my building if he would be willing to do dental blocks for our patients before having facial electrolysis or laser hair removal.

"Linda," responded Dr. Ryan Tennant, "I'll teach you how to do it. It'll just take me a few minutes."

And while I'd never claim to be as skilled as a dentist, I can do a serviceable dental block that takes most of the trauma away from patients undergoing painful upper- and lower-lip hair removal procedures.

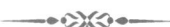

In addition to providing puberty blockers for adolescents, hormone therapy, pre- and postoperative care in gender-confirming surgeries, and trans-friendly aesthetic services, my practice has come to provide primary care for most of our transgender patients. We see cisgender people as well; in fact, I still treat young adults I delivered nearly 30 years ago.

But the point that we provide primary care for transgender patients ranging in age from 5 to 88 years is something that brings me considerable pride and satisfaction.

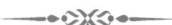

I have found it equally satisfying to share transgender medical information with professional colleagues. All of our staff members are culturally competent and well-versed in transgender care. Our outstanding nurse practitioners provide full transgender care, including anesthetic blocks for hair removal.

I have been lecturing in the area of transgender medicine since about 2011. Since that time, I've participated in every transgender medicine elective course at the University of Washington School of Medicine. I've spoken at Gender Odyssey in Los Angeles and Seattle, the Trans Wellness Conference in Philadelphia, and at First Event in Boston. I have delivered lectures to the University of Washington School of Nursing, the Harborview Residency Program in Emergency Medicine, Physicians' Insurance (my malpractice carrier), the Washington Association of Osteopathic Medicine, the Washington Physician Assistants Association, and even the Annual Dialysis Conference and the northwest chapter of the American Nephrology Nurses Association. In total, this has amounted to over 70 lectures on transgender medicine delivered to healthcare workers.

In recent years, I've heard folks lament that there aren't enough transgender healthcare providers. I couldn't agree more, and there will be *many* more in short order. As it stands, we *do* have outstanding transgender providers who offer a personal sensitivity I can only imagine.

For now, I am grateful to have been present in the somewhat early days of transgender medicine, appreciating and responding to the needs of an amazing community of people. Having worked with the transgender and gender-nonconforming community for 20 years, I'm hoping for 20 more.

With great personal respect for a most resilient community,

— *Linda Gromko, MD*

Queen Anne Medical and Transformative Aesthetics
200 West Mercer #104
Seattle, Washington 98119

Linda@LindaGromkoMD.com
LindaGromkoMD.com (website offering transgender health videos for healthcare professionals)
QueenAnneMedicalAssociates.com (medical practice)

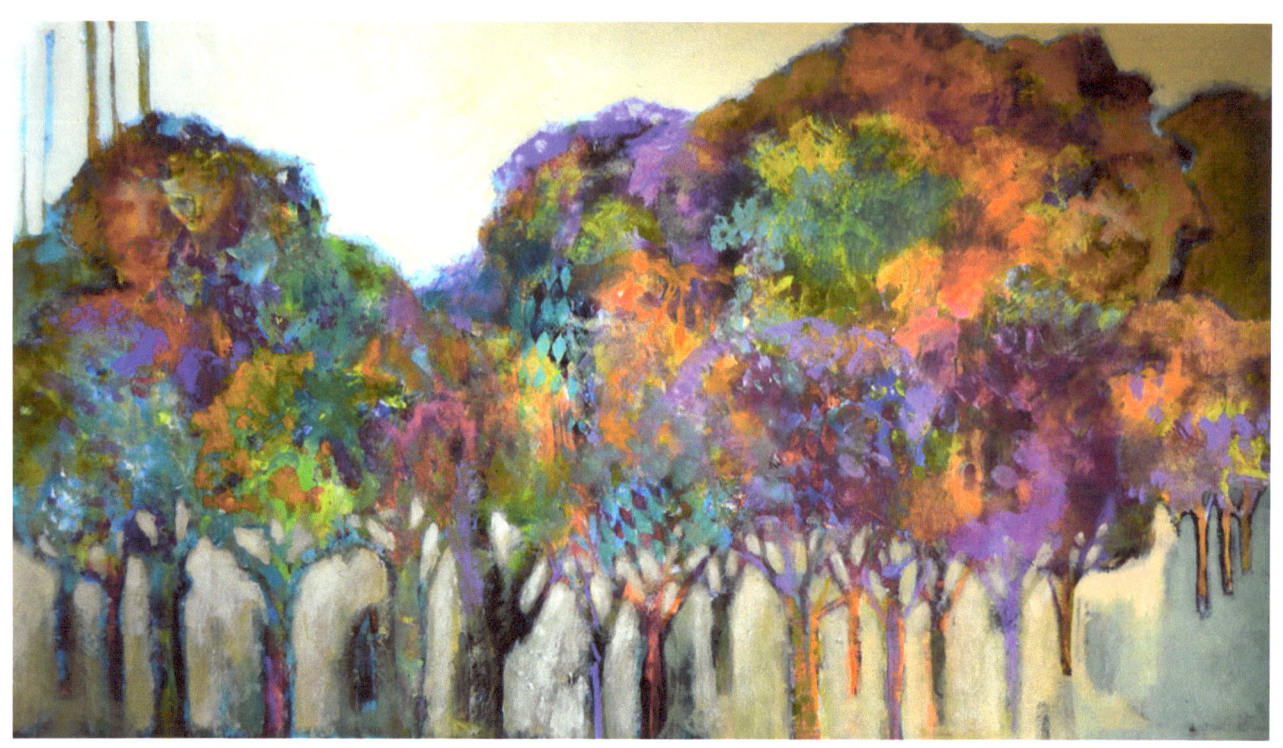

In the Trees

INTRODUCTION

How to Use This Book

If you are reading this book, you are likely examining issues of gender in your life or in the life of someone you care about. Perhaps you have identified as transgender, at least on some level, since you were a small child. Perhaps you were aware of this as simply a feeling that "something was different" for you. Maybe your gender identification has been evolving, becoming clearer as time has passed.

Like many people, you may have begun to realize that being transgender is a real thing and that there are positive steps that can be taken to relieve the gender dysphoria you've experienced. You've known or read about other adults who have transitioned. Or possibly, you have witnessed the transition of teenagers who see the promise of a gender-synchronous life that was only a dream until now.

(For efficiency, I'll be using the term "transgender" throughout this book. Consider this term—for this reading anyway—to represent "transgender and gender-nonconforming.")

I am a board-certified family practice doctor with more than 30 years of experience as a physician, plus two nursing degrees before that. I have worked with the transgender community since 1998, and I have come to value and respect the community enormously.

If you have read my earlier book for trans youth (*Where's MY Book? A Guide for Transgender and Gender Non-Conforming Youth, Their Parents, & Everyone Else*), you will recognize that my writing style is blunt. I rated the earlier book as "R" for "Realistic."

In late 2021, I released *A Practical Reference for Transgender and Gender-Nonconforming Adults*. Because I wrote that book for adults, it went a bit further, maybe an "R-plus." (Genitalia and sexuality were given more prominent roles.) I believe that if we cannot be clear about information, we cannot possibly be effective in sharing the information that counts.

In August 2022, I decided to release *Gender-Affirming Surgeries: Planning through Post-op for Transgender and Gender-Nonconforming Adults* as the stand-alone book you are reading now. It's a slightly modified version of just the surgery content from *A Practical Reference*. (By the way, if you noticed the change from "Gender Non-Conforming" to "Gender-Nonconforming" between my first and most recent books, this is a prefix style update as endorsed by the *Chicago Manual of Style*, not a typing error.)

For most of my practice years, my trans patients needed to travel away from Seattle—out of city, state, or country—to have gender-affirming surgeries. They didn't have the convenience of returning to their surgeon for routine follow-up care. Worse, they did not have the "luxury" of returning to their surgeon if they ran into a problem.

Throughout my career, I have learned that emergency room personnel are highly variable in their biases and knowledge of transgender health. Most professional schools do not offer trans health training at all, although it is changing. But this explains why many healthcare providers don't know how fresh post-op transgender anatomy appears. The ER is the correct place to go when you are experiencing a true life-or-death emergency, and I would never advise a patient to avoid the emergency room. Yet I have seen ER personnel communicate fear or concern when gentle reassurance would have been more—and fully—appropriate. Please refer to Chapter 4 in this book, "In Case of Emergencies."

I have learned from my patients that the postoperative period can seem overwhelming. Forgive me if my reference to delivery is painful, but I remember my postpartum recovery after my son was born: How I voraciously poured over a long-ago book entitled *What Now?* What now, indeed. In spite of years of professional experience in nursing, I felt I knew nothing and that I didn't have a clue on where to start. I was genuinely overwhelmed.

The time after a gender-affirming surgery can feel overwhelming too, and for many compelling reasons:

- You may be hurting or tired.

- You may be frightened that things won't turn out the way you'd imagined.

- You may find that your surgical results look far different from the time-corrected images on the Internet. Time makes an enormous difference when it comes to the normal swelling and bruising that we see immediately post-op. Your results will probably look fine, too—and they normally "remodel" in about six months to a year.

- If you've had genital surgery, your urinary function may require time to adapt. I know that early problems such as a "showerhead" urine stream will usually self-correct. But if you haven't been properly informed that your urinary stream will vary for a while, this can be a source of great concern.

- Your personal support system may be lacking. You may not have people you can turn to for help. By contrast, you may have people who'd gladly help you—but they don't know what to offer, and you may not know what you need.

- Despite all your own preparation and the education provided by your surgical team, you may not know when to worry. So, you worry about everything by default.

- Your usual life difficulties will not automatically disappear postoperatively. You will continue to have normal life responsibilities—with or without surgery.

Please understand that this book is not a substitute for working with your healthcare provider. Your medical situation is unique; your healthcare provider can tailor recommendations specifically to you and your circumstances.

Much of the information in this book may be a review for you; some of the information may be new territory. Some information may apply to you, and some won't. You may certainly disagree with me; let me know if you'd like to discuss something I've written. And please do tell me if you find something that is incorrect or offensive to you.

If you've read my earlier books, you will undoubtedly find repetition and full-on plagiarism from them. Scan this content, or read the book cover to cover, or skip around. Take what is useful for you. Use the book as a springboard from which to formulate new questions and gather more information.

> When describing a gender-affirming surgery to a young client, I said, "Remember, now, this surgery is permanent."
>
> My client responded, "But isn't that the idea?"
>
> Fair enough.
>
> — Linda Gromko, MD

It is important to point out that the decision to pursue a gender-affirming surgery requires careful thought and planning. Most transgender individuals do not have gender-affirming surgeries at all, although the majority of trans individuals state they would want to have them.[2] Some individuals chose one surgery but wouldn't want another. (Many transgender men have top surgery, for example, but may not pursue genital surgery.) Whether or not you have surgery depends on your personal needs and goals, your financial ability to pay or to have insurance pay for surgery, your geographical access to care, and your personal health and life circumstances.

How This Book May Help You

You will find that this book is divided into the following major subject areas:

Chapter 1: Planning for Your Surgery

This chapter helps you examine your surgical goals, such as optimizing your health in preparation for surgery (including health screening, smoking cessation, and weight management), paying for your surgery and related expenses, choosing the surgeon who is best for you, and getting the letters that are required to have surgery. We examine the critical six weeks before surgery with respect to your home and work situations, and we discuss making arrangements for postoperative help.

Chapter 2: Feminizing Surgeries

This chapter explains facial feminization surgeries, breast augmentation, and body contouring for feminization. Vaginoplasty is covered in detail, including penile-inversion vaginoplasty, penile-inversion vaginoplasty with labiaplasty done later, the zero-depth or limited-depth vaginoplasty, and the newer peritoneal pull-through vaginoplasty. Colon procedures, including the rectosigmoid colon and right-colon surgeries, are discussed, as are new developments in using tilapia grafts to construct the vaginal canal.

Chapter 3: Masculinizing Surgeries

Here we cover facial masculinization surgeries, gender-affirming chest reconstruction (top surgery), hysterectomy and bilateral salpingo-oophorectomy, and vaginectomy.

---

2 "In the most robust survey to date, 25% of TGNB respondents report having undergone some form of gender confirming surgery." Ian T. Nolan, Christopher J. Kuhner, and Geolani W. Dy, "Demographic and Temporal Trends in Transgender Identities and Gender Confirming Surgery," *Translational Andrology and Urology* 8, no. 3 (June 2019): 186, doi: 10.21037/tau.2019.04.09.

Choosing the correct genital surgery according to individual surgical goals is covered in detail. Current genital surgeries include metoidioplasty and metoidioplasty with urethral extension. Phalloplasty techniques discussed include the radial forearm flap phalloplasty, the anterior lateral thigh flap phalloplasty, and the delayed pedicle flap phalloplasty. Construction of the glans penis (glansplasty) and two types of erectile devices are covered. Gender nonbinary surgeries, including penis-preserving vaginoplasty and gender nullification surgeries, are discussed.

Chapter 4: In Case of Emergencies

While serious, life-threatening complications are rare, it is important to be able to recognize when you are in medical trouble and how to get the urgent care you need. This section covers situations where you may have to call 911, as well as less emergent circumstances.

Chapter 5: Taking Care of Yourself after Surgery

We review the general flow of what happens in the hospital or surgical center. Home care covers setting up systems with the people who support you, as well as optimizing your bedroom area for a comfortable recovery. This chapter discusses pain management, nutrition (especially fluid management and protein intake), and the basics of dressing changes and wound care. We also cover recognizing signs of depression that may appear during the post-op period.

Chapter 6: Specific Postoperative Circumstances Dealing with Specific Surgeries

Vaginal dilation is reviewed, as are pointers for recognizing urinary variations and urinary tract infections and managing and avoiding constipation. Detailed information is included regarding top surgery and the several variations of phalloplasty. The chapter offers information on penile tattoos to enhance phalloplasty and includes an interview with a manager of Quest House recovery facility. The chapter also covers products that assist with recovery in feminizing, masculinizing, and nonbinary surgeries.

This summary would imply that this book covers everything! But do understand that it was never intended to be the "only reference you'll ever need." There are whole segments of information that have not been included, not because they aren't important, but because the field is so broad that there is simply far too much to cover.

All this information is provided with the intention that you individually will be more likely to have a better experience and outcome if you are armed with information. If you're a family member or healthcare provider, perhaps this information will help you advocate more powerfully for your friend, partner, offspring, or client.

Know that this book has drawn from a host of contributors: physicians who were kind enough to review the book for accuracy, my years of clinical practice with the transgender and gender-nonconforming community, and the stories and helpful gems of personal advice from willing clients.

I wish you the very best in your journey and hope that this book will help you along the way.

—*Linda Gromko, MD*

Challenges with Online Links and Internet References

Even though all online links to reference citations and websites were checked and current at the time of the book's printing, some may no be longer available. And if we've linked to a periodical reference, the reference may have changed. What to do?

- Try entering the title or topic in the search bar of your browser.
- If an address of a link is spread out over two lines, you may have to type in the whole link to get it to work.

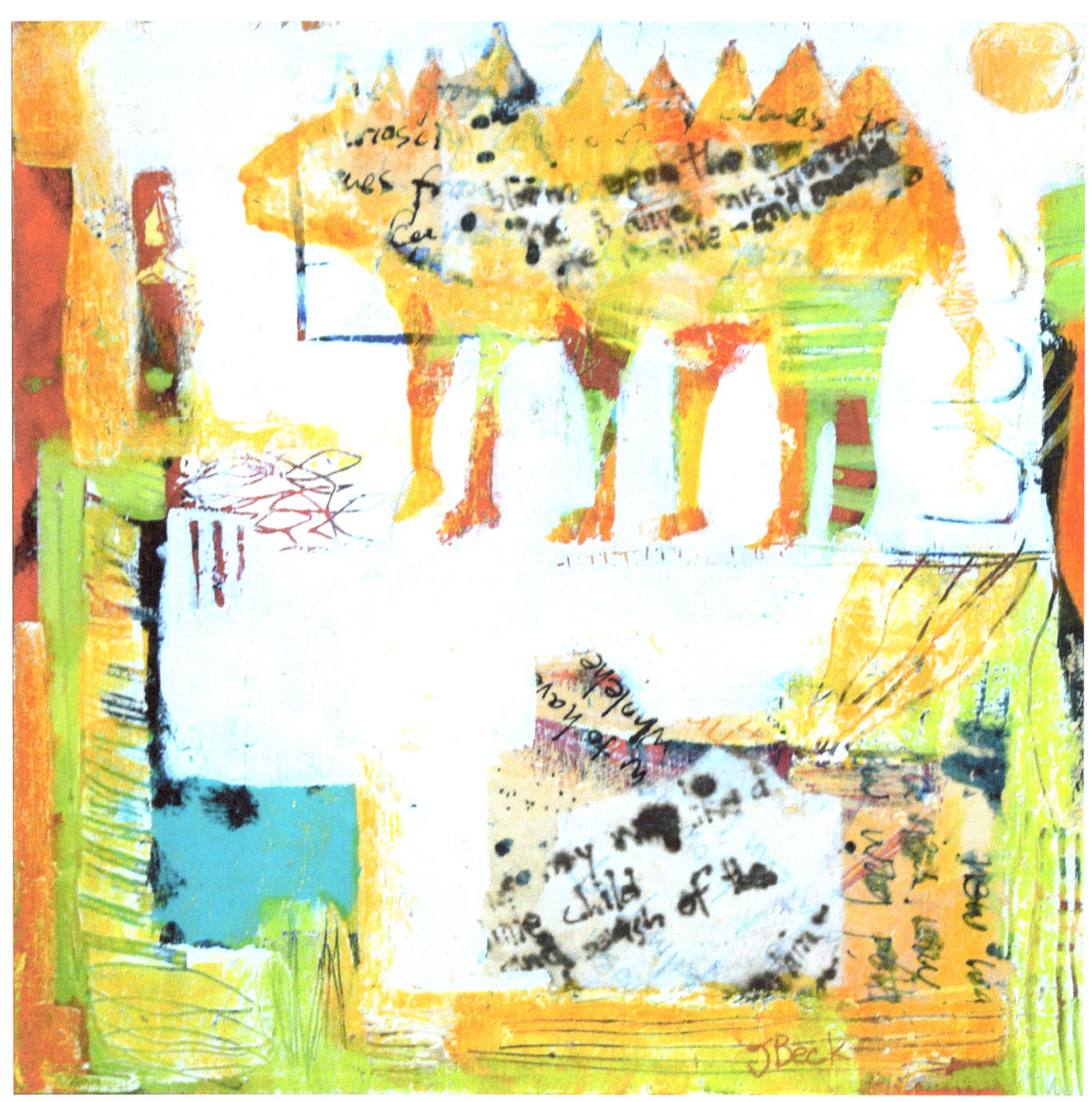

Many Socks

CHAPTER 1
Planning for Your Surgery

Waiting for Your Gender-Affirming Surgery

If you wish to have your gender-affirming surgery performed by one of the country's better-known surgeons, you may have to be on a waiting list for **2 to 3 years**. You can cancel, of course, but you may forfeit your deposit.

And you can ask to be on a cancellation list—that is, to be moved up in line if someone ahead of you cancels. **Fortunately, these prolonged waiting times have lessened as more surgeons have become expert in transgender surgeries.**

The Critical 1 to 2 Years before Surgery

Orchestrating a gender-affirming surgery would challenge the most skilled of project managers. The year or two before surgery is a busy time with much to accomplish and important consequences if details are missed.

In my experience as a clinician, patients undergo a range of emotions in the year or two prior to their surgeries: excitement, frustration, confusion, anxiety, relief, a sense of feeling overwhelmed—you name it. It's all understandable. Arranging and having surgery is a complicated process, and available support is inconsistent at best. If you don't have a therapy relationship already established, this may be a great time to develop one. You'll likely need a therapist to write a supportive letter required for surgery anyway.

Gender-affirming surgery is a major decision. Surgeries are expensive, insurance coverage is variable, and outcomes are never guaranteed (although they are remarkable in most cases). Surgical results are, for the most part, irreversible. That is to say, the only possible way back from a surgical outcome you don't like may be to have more surgery. **And, if insurance doesn't cover a procedure, it may or may not cover a complication or reversal.**

Let's look at some of the factors you will want to consider before having a gender-affirming surgery. Use this chapter as a surgery planner or workbook. Check off what you've already accomplished and make notes as to your questions and to-do items.

Your Personal Goals

What Do You Hope Your Surgery Will Accomplish?

Define your goals as precisely as you can. Examine the detailed descriptions of the various surgeries to assure that you are on the right track. You're more likely to get what you want if you know precisely what it *is* that you want.

How Realistic Are Your Hopes and Expectations?

Arrange for an in-person consultation with your surgeon, or an introductory Skype consultation if you live far away (see "Choosing Your Surgeon" on pages 16–20). After getting to know you better, your surgeon should ask you to define your desired goals of the surgery as precisely as you can. Photos are often helpful. Then ask for an honest and realistic assessment: Can the surgeon deliver the results you are requesting? Everyone comes to the operating room with different "raw materials." One person may require more or different surgeries to achieve the desired results. Don't be afraid to get a second opinion. Experienced surgeons welcome them and are not offended by your wanting a second opinion.

Q When is gender-affirming surgery required?

A That's a question that only you can answer for yourself. Most trans people never have surgery at all, although 75 percent of transgender women say they would want it.[3]

In working with trans men and women, I often ask, "If money and family were not factors, what would your surgical goals be?" Or alternatively, "If you were completely alone on an isolated island yet somehow had access to gender-affirming surgery, what type of surgery would you have? Would you have surgery at all?"

If You Are Envisioning Multiple Surgeries, Where Will You Start?

Are you planning a surgery such as phalloplasty that requires several steps to achieve the results you need? Different surgeons do the stages in an order based on their experience and preferences. Know the recommended sequence of your surgeries; again, this will require a consultation with the surgeon.

Which surgery is most important to you? Is a large Adam's apple interfering with your comfort in the world? If so, a tracheal shave may be more important than a breast augmentation or rhinoplasty.

---

[3] Per the 2010 *National Transgender Discrimination Survey Report on Health and Health Care*: "Most survey respondents had sought or accessed some form of transition-related care. Counseling and hormone treatment were notably more utilized than any surgical procedures, although the majority reported wanting to "someday" be able to have surgery … Three-quarters of transgender women reported that they desired to have surgery at some point in the future or had already done so. However, it is impossible to know how many would desire or utilize surgery if it were more financially accessible … Genital surgery, on the other hand, remains out of reach for a large majority, despite being desired by most respondents." Jaime M. Grant et al., *National Transgender Discrimination Survey Report on Health and Health Care* (Washington DC: National Center for Transgender Equality, 2010), 10–11, 16, https://cancer-network.org/wp-content/uploads/2017/02/National_Transgender_Discrimination_Survey_Report_on_health_and_health_care.pdf.

> I'll say, "Imagine yourself in an emergency room or a nursing home. Would you be okay with your genitalia in those situations?" If you are embarrassed or ashamed of your genitalia in a medical situation, this is something to consider. Your viewpoint may also change with age.
>
> — *Marci Bowers, MD*

Are Your Goals Reachable by Surgery?

Realistically examine with your healthcare provider, your partner, your therapist, or anyone you trust whether surgical treatment even applies to you. Suppose you are seeking to feminize your appearance and feel that your outward presentation is more important than your genital appearance. If so, you may elect facial feminization surgery and perhaps breast augmentation. Genital surgery may not be something you want or need. Except in medical treatment or intimate sexual contact with a partner, who really sees our genitals anyway? (The obvious answer is that *we* do, and genital dysphoria can be severe enough to prompt vaginoplasty or phalloplasty well before outward presentation is addressed.)

Do the Collective Benefits of Surgery Outweigh the Risks for You?

Everyone has their own risk tolerance. All surgeries have risks and you will get a better idea of what these may be as you read the details of respective surgeries in Chapter 2. Only you can make this assessment. Although serious complications are uncommon, would you regret having surgery if you did have a serious complication? Or would you look at the surgery as something that simply had to be done, and manage problems if they arose?

Optimizing Your Personal Health before Surgery

During the 1 to 2 years prior to your surgery, compile information about your own health. This is the time to take stock of your own medical fitness. Here are some things to consider.

Get a Thorough Medical Evaluation

Your healthcare provider will take a medical history and perform a physical exam. Ask for lab tests that reflect your body's level of functioning.

Laboratory Tests for a General Evaluation

Here is a list of commonly ordered blood tests. Ask your healthcare provider which tests might apply to you.

- **CBC (complete blood count)** assures us that your bone marrow is producing normal red blood cells, white blood cells, and platelets. This test can indicate anemia and variation in red cell size.

- **CMP (comprehensive metabolic profile)** measures your blood sugar, kidney and liver function, electrolytes (sodium, potassium, etc.), and reflects your body's acid and base balance.

- **TSH (thyroid stimulating hormone)** is the pituitary hormone that regulates production of thyroid hormone in the thyroid gland. The thyroid hormone regulates your metabolic rate—or how your body uses energy. A high TSH is associated with low thyroid function.

- **Lipid panel** measures your cholesterol level and may signal indicators that place a person at higher risk for cardiovascular disease.

- **HbA1c (hemoglobin A1c or glycosylated hemoglobin)** reflects your blood sugar level during the prior 3 months and may suggest diabetes if it is elevated. It is also used to monitor how well a diabetic is managing their blood sugar.

- **STI (STD) profile** screens for sexually transmitted infections, which used to be called sexually transmitted diseases (I generally include HIV, tests for hepatitis B and hepatitis C, syphilis, herpes simplex type 1 and type 2, gonorrhea, and chlamydia).

- **PSA (prostate specific antigen)** for AMAB individuals age 50 and over.

- **Estradiol and free and total testosterone levels.**

Other Medical Conditions to Be Evaluated before Surgery

- **Make a list of your own ongoing medical issues or concerns—essentially, a "problem list."**
  Your healthcare provider does this routinely. Do your lists agree?

- **Do you have diabetes, heart disease, asthma, depression, systemic skin disease (such as psoriasis) or other conditions that might impact your surgery?**
  If so, get everything "tuned up," so you will be in the best medical condition possible before your surgery. Ask your primary care provider about this perhaps even before you consult your surgeon.

- **Are there specific health benchmarks you must achieve prior to surgery?**
  If so, nail these down now. For example, if you are a diabetic, your surgeon may require a specific hemoglobin A1c level. The HbA1c reflects your blood sugar over the prior 3 months. A normal HbA1c will run under 5.6 percent; as a diabetic, your HbA1c will likely run higher. Your surgeon,

however, may require that you must have a HbA1c of 7.0 or under to qualify for surgery. (A newer way to assess blood sugar is the "time within range," or the portion of time during which your blood sugar is in a normal range. This eliminates the evening-out effect of high and low blood sugars in the HbA1c.) Check to see what *your* surgeon requires and get your blood sugar under good control now—not just for surgery, but for the rest of your life.

- **If you have a heart condition, your primary care provider and your surgeon may ask your cardiologist to clear you prior to surgery.**
  This process may include a cardiologist's examination, a current electrocardiogram (EKG), a cholesterol (lipid) panel, and an echocardiogram to evaluate your heart valves, and your heart's ejection fraction (that is, the "squeeze" function of your heart).

  It's very reasonable to have a presurgical cardiology evaluation if you are a diabetic. It is commonly believed that diabetics have a higher risk for cardiovascular disease.[4]

  If your primary care doctor hears a heart murmur that hasn't been heard or evaluated before, see a cardiologist. (I remember a patient who had a new—and loud—murmur when I performed her preoperative exam. She was found to have a serious mitral valve problem. Her facial feminization surgery was rescheduled; she had to wait for a year after her heart valve was repaired.)

> A patient of mine had had a heart attack a couple of years before she scheduled her sexual reassignment surgery in Thailand. She declined the cardiology evaluation I had recommended. When she got to Thailand, though, her surgeon required that she have the same evaluation I had recommended. Thankfully, she passed inspection and had a successful surgery. But suppose she hadn't passed her tests? She would have traveled a long distance only to have her surgery denied. Worse, she might have had a serious cardiac event, cardiac surgery, or death far away from home.
>
> — *Linda Gromko, MD*

- **Are you up-to-date on generally recommended screening tests, such as colonoscopy screening for colon cancer, a Pap test for cervical cancer, a PSA for prostate cancer, or mammogram screening for breast cancer?**
  Screening is often a controversial topic; the USPSTF (**uspreventiveservicestaskforce.org/uspstf**) publishes recommendations as dictated by evidence-based medicine. Have a discussion with your healthcare provider now about how these recommendations may apply to you. Suppose you found something concerning on a screening test? Take care of it now so there won't be surprises later.

---

[4] New research questions commonly held beliefs vis-à-vis cardiovascular risk assessment in patients with diabetes: "Diabetes has long been considered a 'cardiovascular risk equivalent.' This statement was formerly based in the Finnish study, in which T2DM patients without coronary heart disease (CHD) events showed a similar coronary mortality as nondiabetic patients who had a previous coronary event…[however] Recent evidences indicate that CHD risk in T2DM is not universally similar to the risk of patients with prior cardiovascular disease, but is highly heterogeneous… Type 2 diabetes increases cardiovascular risk in 2 to fourfold, but cannot be considered a risk equivalent due to the high heterogeneity." Marcello Casaccia Bertoluci and Viviane Zorzanelli Rocha, "Cardiovascular Risk Assessment in Patients with Diabetes," *Diabetology & Metabolic Syndrome* 9, no. 25 (April 20, 2017), https://doi.org/10.1186/s13098-017-0225-1.

- Do you have a blood clotting problem that may increase your risk of a blood clot in your legs or in your lungs after surgery? A venous thromboembolism (VTE) or deep vein thrombosis (DVT) can travel to the lung where it is called a pulmonary embolism (PE).

  Both conditions are serious; a pulmonary embolism (resulting from a DVT that travels to the lungs) can be fatal. Surgeries carry an increased risk for blood clots in the perioperative period (the time around surgery). Know if you have a condition that increases your personal risk and get your plan in order. For example, **if you've had a prior VTE, DVT, or PE, you may have already been evaluated by a hematologist (blood specialist) to see if you have a "hypercoagulable state."**

A hypercoagulable state is a condition that increases your clotting risk. If you have a predisposition to blood clots (also called a thrombophilia) or have had a clot before, your surgeon will want you to consult a hematologist prior to surgery. This doesn't necessarily disqualify you from having surgery. But your surgeon and you can make a management plan well ahead of time (that is, using low-molecular-weight heparin at the time of surgery).

Your surgeon will want you to see a hematologist if you currently take an anticoagulant medication for any reason or have done so in the past.

Again, this is not an automatic disqualifier, but you and your surgeon will want a perioperative anticoagulant plan to keep you safe. Here are examples of common anticoagulant medications:

- **Heparin**
  Used in an IV (intravenous) form in patients being treated for a DVTs or PEs; more commonly used in years past.

- **Low-molecular-weight heparin (Lovanox)**
  Used as a subcutaneous injection twice a day to treat DVTs or PEs. Sometimes used during surgery to prevent a DVT or PE.

- **Warfarin (Coumadin)**
  An older but less expensive oral anticoagulant used in DVTs, PEs, atrial fibrillation, and so on. Serum levels must be carefully monitored; warfarin interacts with many medications and foods that can move a person's blood clotting indicators out of a therapeutic window. Too little medication, and clots form more easily; too much, and patients can have life-threatening bleeding.

- **DOACs (direct oral anticoagulants)**
  These more expensive newer agents are taken orally in the treatment of DVTs, PEs, atrial fibrillation, and so on. Monitoring of blood levels are not required as with warfarin. There are many available, such as apixaban (Eliquis), rivaroxaban (Xarelto), and dabigatran (Pradaxa).

If you are currently taking an anticoagulant for *therapeutic* reasons (that is, to treat a recent blood clot or because you have recently had a coronary artery stent placed), you may be advised to postpone your surgery until later. This is not automatic but be sure that everyone on your surgical and medical teams agree that this is a safe time for your surgery to be performed.

> Most anticoagulant therapies can be managed by stopping the oral medications and using a Lovanox bridge without having bleeding problems in surgery. This is obviously done in coordination with a patient's hematologist or cardiologist.
>
> — *Toby Meltzer, MD*

- **Are there any other medical conditions that might be prudently evaluated before surgery?**
  Suppose you have a family history or personal history of kidney, urinary tract, or liver disease. Perhaps a physician has recommended you have further evaluation. Now is the time, *before your gender-affirming surgery*, to complete these specialist evaluations.

Modify Any Personal Health Habits That May Impact Your Surgical Risks

Now is the ideal time to examine your personal health habits. Modify any behaviors that might make it more dangerous to have a surgery and recover without complications.

Stop Smoking Now If You Smoke (Tobacco, Marijuana, Hookahs) or Use Tobacco Products

Your surgeon will advise you that smoking impairs your capacity to heal and increases your risk of blood clots. Most surgeons will not perform surgery on you if you smoke. (They'll test your urine before surgery and will cancel your operation if you have been smoking.)

At the second annual WPATH Live Surgery Training course in February–March 2019, several surgeons recommended quitting smoking 3 to 4 weeks before surgery and abstaining until 3 to 4 weeks after. (Better yet, take this opportunity to quit for good.)

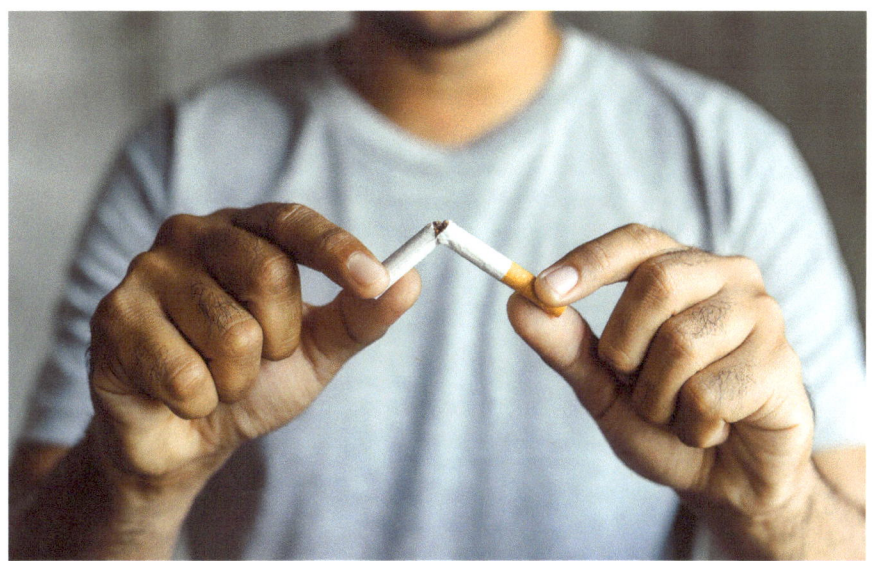

Help with Quitting Smoking

Quitting smoking isn't easy. In fact, nicotine is thought to be as addictive as heroin and cocaine.* But you must stop all forms of tobacco use before surgery. While most people quit cold turkey, there are some powerful pharmacologic agents to help you quit:

- **Nicotine patches** (NicoDerm) and **nicotine gum** (Nicorette) are available without a prescription. These agents occupy nicotine receptors in your brain to help you wean off the nicotine in cigarettes. Some people claim that vaping nicotine may help them transition off other tobacco products; we really don't know this, and we are generally advising that people avoid vaping—particularly in the setting of COVID-19.

    Be alert that all these nicotine replacement products will cause vasoconstriction (constriction of the blood vessels) and impair your ability to heal. In addition, nicotine changes your carboxy-hemoglobin receptors, allowing carbon monoxide to attach to your hemoglobin molecules more easily than oxygen. Plus, they will show up on a urine test. So, use them to help you stop smoking, but stop all nicotine products several weeks ahead of your surgery.

- **Bupropion** (Wellbutrin) is a prescribed antidepressant that shows excellent efficacy in reducing cravings for cigarettes. It is marketed under the name of Zyban for this purpose. If you struggle with depression, you may experience a double benefit in that the medication may help you stop smoking and alleviate your depression as well.

- **Chantix** (varenicline) is also prescribed specifically for smoking cessation. When a person smokes tobacco, the nicotine from cigarettes occupies nicotinic acetylcholine receptors in the brain. This causes the release of dopamine, which we knew as the "drugs, sex, and rock 'n' roll" neurotransmitter in medical school. The release of dopamine in the brain contributes to an overall sense of well-being.

    When Chantix is used, it occupies the nicotine receptors so that the nicotine from smoking cannot occupy them. This in turn results in less dopamine, providing the overall sense of well-being so smoking doesn't have the same effect it used to. While Chantix doesn't work for everyone, I've had some great results with my patients who've used it. Chantix gives the user a clearly outlined path to quitting. Plus, you do not quit on the first day but rather in a few days or weeks into the course. **

    Pfizer, the maker of Chantix, has discontinued an earlier black box warning cautioning users to report psychiatric symptoms such as mood changes, hostility, agitation, and suicidal ideation. Be alert, nonetheless.

---

* Vanessa Caceres, "9 Best Ways to Quit Smoking," *US News & World Report*, last reviewed February 12, 2021, https://health.usnews.com/wellness/articles/best-ways-to-quit-smoking.

** Per the Chantix (Varenicline) label: "Approaches to selecting a tobacco quit date: May either choose a fixed quit date (i.e., start varenicline, then quit on day 8) or a flexible quit date (i.e., start varenicline, then quit between days 8 to 35). Alternatively, a gradual quit date (i.e., start varenicline and reduce smoking 50% by week 4, reduce an additional 50% by week 8, and continue reducing with a goal of complete abstinence by week 12) is acceptable (Hajek 2011; Rigotti 2020; manufacturer's labeling)." Please see drugs.com/ppa/varenicline.html.

> Chantix is a more expensive medication than bupropion; insurance may not cover it or they may require that you try bupropion first.
>
> Here are some other tools:
>
> - Hypnotherapy helps many people quit smoking.
>
> - 1-800-QUIT-NOW (1-800-784-8669) is a phone number that directs you to Quit Smoking programs in your locale.
>
> - *Allen Carr's Easy Way to Quit Smoking Without Willpower* (November 2019) is a useful book that has helped many of my patients. As with Chantix, Carr doesn't recommend that you stop smoking immediately. Rather, he walks you through the process, preparing you to stop. I've seen his approach work for people who've chain-smoked for decades. Find it online.

When you do quit, quit for good. If you slip, recognize that it happens and quit again. As your life gets better, don't shorten it with a technicality like a smoking-related disease.

Manage Your Weight

If you are overweight or obese, your surgeon will advise you what BMI (body mass index) you must have to qualify for surgery.

- **The BMI is a measurement based on height and weight alone.**
  It has nothing to do with gender. You can Google "BMI calculator" and enter your height and weight to find your own BMI. A BMI of over 30 means you are technically obese; if your BMI is over 40, you are severely obese (formerly and rudely called "morbidly obese") or at least 100 pounds above your ideal body weight. Obesity increases your risk of adverse events occurring during surgery as well as your risk of poor wound healing.

- **Learn now what BMI is specified by your surgeon.**
  That way, you'll have a reasonable time to lose weight before surgery. Certainly, there can be some leeway with a BMI measure. For example, if you are muscular from working out, your BMI will be higher than that of a sedentary person with less muscle. Muscle simply weighs more than fat tissue, and a slightly higher BMI in a well-muscled individual may not increase surgical risk.

  The point is that you need to know the standard set by your surgeon. At the second annual WPATH Live Surgery Training course in February–March 2019, I heard BMI limits of 32 to 35, but several surgeons said they did top surgery on severely obese transmasculine individuals. BMI requirements may vary between vaginoplasty, phalloplasty, and chest reconstruction, and genital surgeries have more stringent requirements. Again, find out your surgeon's requirements and be mindful that surgeons set these standards out of concern for your good outcome.

Help with Weight Loss

Just as with stopping smoking, try to lose weight for good, not just for surgery.

Here are some tips we compiled during a weight loss support group we ran in our practice and others from the National Weight Control Registry (NWCR) (nwcr.ws). The NWCR is helpful, as it tracks the habits of people who have lost a significant amount of weight (66 pounds) and kept it off for a significant time (5.5 years).

- Plan to do some exercise nearly every day; walking is the most popular among long-term members of National Weight Control Registry.
- Eat breakfast regularly.
- Limit TV watching to 10 hours per week.
- The best exercise for you is the one you'll actually do.
- Plan your eating and record your daily food intake.
- Drink water freely.
- Limit alcohol; think of alcohol as having calories without nutritional value.
- Focus on fresh vegetables and fruit (nobody gains weight from carrots) and lean protein.
- Limit, but don't eliminate, treats.
- You may choose to eat "normally" on weekends, for example. But realize that like most of us, you may not have eaten "normally" before.
- Use smaller-size plates; you'll eat less.
- Be realistic: "The best way to lose 10 pounds is to lose 5."
- Weigh yourself at regular intervals and keep track of your progress. Made it to your goal? Use a margin of 2 pounds; if you're up 2 pounds, get back to work!

- **If you need to lose a moderate amount of weight, consider Weight Watchers or Noom.**
  Weight Watchers is logical, easy to do, and flexible, plus it can be done online. If you haven't done the program for a while, there have been many recent changes (weightwatchers.com). Noom is quite new and features online and group participation (noom.com).

- **Look at Kathy Abascal's To Quiet Inflammation plan (tqidiet.com).**
  Abascal focuses on portion balance: two-thirds of any size plate is for vegetables and fruit, and no more than one-sixth of the plate is for protein or whole grains. She conducts in-person and online classes. It's a reasonable approach to healthy eating; many followers of the plan report that they lose weight and have fewer symptoms attributable to inflammation, such as skin rashes, joint aching, and bowel irritability.

- **Search for information on the Mediterranean diet for weight loss or maintenance.**

- **If your BMI is over 40 and you have already tried every conceivable way to control your weight, consult a bariatric surgeon.**
  Most people trying gastric bypass surgeries will lose around 100 pounds. There *are* people who learn to "eat around" the constraints of a gastric bypass and gain the weight back. But it may be the most successful route to controlling weight-related conditions such as diabetes and its many complications, degenerative joint disease, and certain cardiopulmonary conditions.[5]

Address Your Alcohol Intake

Excessive alcohol use can complicate your surgical and postoperative course. Be honest with your surgeon about how much alcohol you use, and tell your surgeon if you have alcohol withdrawal symptoms when you stop drinking (shaking, tremors, fever, DTs, hallucinations, and so on). Certainly, it's best to get the use of alcohol other recreational substances under control now if they represent problems for you.

Know Your STI (STD) Status

If you know you have HIV or another blood-borne sexually transmitted infection such as hepatitis B or C, tell your surgeon for their protection. (Of course, all healthcare providers use universal precautions to prevent themselves from becoming infected, but I think disclosing this information is a simple courtesy.) If you are concerned that you may be infected, find out now so you can be completely assessed prior to surgery.

Allow at Least a Year for Hair Removal If Your Surgeon Requires Hair Removal for Genital Surgery (Vaginoplasty or Phalloplasty)

One of my clients recommends 18 months to 2 years for phalloplasty hair removal. Why is this necessary? We can see hair growing in the neovagina postoperatively, as the scrotum is used to construct the vagina. (Is hair in the vagina world-ending? Probably not, but it's hardly the desired outcome. It can also cause odor, irritation, and decreased vaginal depth if a clump of hair rests in the vaginal vault.)

Q If some of my genital hair grows back, does it mean I had poor treatments?

A Not necessarily; there are simply *so* many hairs there, including hairs under the surface that may not have been visible during treatment.

With phalloplasty, hair must be removed from the donor site (such as the forearm, anterior lateral thigh, or back). If it is not removed, hair may grow on the outside of the phallus, or worse, inside the urethra where it is even more difficult to remove. Hair in the urethra can be dense enough to reduce the flow of urine or cause postvoid dribbling. The hair can also react with urine to form tiny concretions that reduce urine flow. Be sure to check with your surgeon to see which method of hair removal (such as electrolysis versus laser) they prefer. Know also that not all surgeons require hair removal prior to vaginoplasty.

---

5   Maurizio De Luca et al., "Indications for Surgery for Obesity and Weight-Related Diseases: Position Statements from the International Federation for the Surgery of Obesity and Metabolic Disorders (IFSO)," *Obesity Surgery* 26, no. 8 (July 2016): 1659–96, https://doi.org/10.1007/s11695-016-2271-4.

> Dr. Richard Santucci cautions that 2 years of hair removal may serve as a barrier for people seeking phalloplasty. He encourages people to do several cycles of hair removal, but not to delay surgery to get a year or two of electrolysis completed. He reports seeing some hair growth occurring even with conscientious removal.

Optimize Your Physical Fitness

It makes sense that a physically fit body can respond to the stresses of surgery and recovery with greater resilience. You don't have to be a jock, but do get some daily physical exercise, even if it's simply walking. Exercise also increases your collateral circulation: extra blood vessels grow to bring more blood to an area, which is particularly important for phalloplasties.

Check Your Immunization Status

Check your immunizations, particularly if you have a chronic illness (such as diabetes, heart disease, or asthma) or if you are traveling out of the country for surgery. You will be expected to update your immunizations as you get closer to surgery. It's not a "one-and-done" matter.

Paying for Your Surgery

Gender-affirming surgeries are expensive. While insurance coverage varies, it is more common than ever to find that gender-affirming surgeries are covered. Larger employers, particularly tech companies, have been leaders in gender-inclusive coverage. Examples include Microsoft, Google, Facebook, Amazon, Boeing, and Starbucks. Many government-funded organizations, such as the University of Washington, the State of Washington, and the City of Seattle, cover gender-affirming surgeries. A variety of other municipalities do also, such as San Francisco, Berkeley, and San Jose.

That said, if you are looking for a job, why *not* share your skills and talents with an employer that fully supports you as an individual? As of this writing, Washington State's Apple Care through the Health Care Authority and Medicare cover gender-affirming surgeries, although their reimbursement may be so low as to limit the number of surgeons who participate.

- The point of the above is to advise you to carefully check your own health insurance before making any assumptions. When you contact your health insurance company, use the customer service contact information on your insurance card but also ask to speak with a representative who deals with transgender coverage. You may save yourself time, frustration, and misinformation. Insurance may cover presurgical hair removal, so ask!

- Read your insurance plan carefully. You are generally responsible for paying the deductible amount specified by the plan. Then you may have to pay a percentage of the surgery cost.

- If you have an accountant, check to see what noncovered surgical or presurgical expenses (such as hair removal) you may declare for tax purposes.

- If you have a health savings account or a cafeteria plan available as a benefit from your employer, you may be able to use pretax dollars to pay for your portion of a gender-affirming surgery.[6]

Find a Trans-Advocacy Legal Organization to Help You Understand Your Insurance and Get Your Surgery Covered

When attorney Noah Lewis was a student at Harvard Law School, he was able to get his *own* gender-affirming surgery covered, although it had been previously excluded from the Harvard policy. Lewis went on to establish the nonprofit organization Transcend Legal with the aim of helping others get insurance approval for gender-affirming care by appealing adverse decisions and overcoming roadblocks. Lewis produced an informative video series to help individuals understand and navigate the health insurance maze. While Transcend Legal has closed, you can still find Lewis's video series on YouTube (youtube.com/channel/UC8ufMm0N1n3JjRpJtAuGgPA/playlists).

Noah Lewis is now affiliated with the Transgender Legal Defense and Education Fund, a 501(c)(3) nonprofit organization "committed to ending discrimination based upon gender identity and expression and to achieving equality for transgender people through public education, test-case litigation, direct legal services, and public policy efforts." While the organization deals with a variety of trans discrimination issues, individuals wishing information regarding insurance denials may contact TLDEF at tldef.org.

Surgery Itself Is Only *One* Expense

Remember that the cost of surgery itself represents only a portion of the cost of having surgery. Here are some other expenses that you may incur that are unlikely to be covered by insurance:

- **Living expenses for the time of surgery, the time off for recovery, and postoperative visits.**

  - You may buy more prepared or take-out food.

  - You may pay someone to help you with cleaning or personal care.

  - You may have expenses for items such as wound dressings, pads, or other items you use postoperatively.

  - You may incur rideshare expenses such as Uber, Lyft, or a taxi if you are unable to drive for a while.

- **Travel expenses for yourself (and a travel partner) if your surgeon is not local.**

  - You may have to stay in a hotel or Airbnb when you are not in the hospital. Your travel partner will have additional room and board expenses while your meals and so on are covered in the hospital.

  - If you have a complication after returning home from surgery, it may be difficult to find a local surgeon willing or qualified to help you. Consider having a reserve for extra expenses of traveling back to your original surgeon if additional surgery is needed.

---

6   "Transition-related medical care is eligible with consumer-directed healthcare accounts, which was a result of the United States Tax Court's 2010 decision in *O'Donnabhain v. Commissioner* which ruled that a transgender woman's medical expenses for hormone therapy and sex reassignment surgery were legitimate treatments for GID and therefore tax-deductible under Federal law. As a result of this pivotal court decision, on November 21, 2011, the Internal Revenue Service (IRS) affirmed that transgender people can deduct the costs of hormone therapy and sex reassignment surgery from their gross income as medical expenses for the treatment of gender identity disorder (GID)." FSA Store, "Transgender Counseling or Surgery: FSA Eligibility," accessed July 28, 2021, https://fsastore.com/FSA-Eligibility-List/T/Transgender-Counseling-or-Surgery-E717.aspx.

- If you are planning to travel out of the country, are there country-specific costs that you might expect? (Don't forget to get immunized prior to leaving the country if this is appropriate. For that matter, update your immunizations even if your surgeon is only a block away.)

- Additional costs for people who depend on your income, such as childcare costs.

Other Ways to Help Cover Surgical and Nonsurgical Costs (Besides Insurance)

You may have to be creative here, and you may not have great options. But here are some options my patients have used:

- **Benefits from an employer.**
  If you have a health savings account or a cafeteria plan available as a benefit from your employer, you may be able to use pretax dollars to pay for your portion of a gender-affirming surgery.[7]

- **Tax benefits.**
  If you have an accountant, check to see what noncovered surgical or presurgical expenses (such as hair removal, travel, and medical supplies) you may declare for tax purposes. This saves you money, but after the fact. Save receipts so you can deduct these costs.

- **Military veterans and active duty personnel.**
  When President Donald Trump tweeted a ban on transgender military service on July 26, 2017, surgeon Dr. Christine McGinn countered that she would offer gender-reassignment surgery pro bono for active duty military personnel. Dr. McGinn confirmed that her Papillon Center (drchristinemcginn.com) offers a 15 percent discount on surgical fees for veterans and that she provides pro bono surgery for active duty military personnel.[8] Dr. McGinn, a former Navy flight surgeon, stated in her CNN interview, "If the commander-in-chief won't take care of our veterans, our veterans will." Watch the interview in its entirety at cnn.com/videos/tv/2017/07/29/trans-ex-navy-surgeon-on-trumps-ban.cnn.

  On June 19, 2021, the Department of Veterans Affairs announced a reversal of this ban and that gender-affirmation surgery will be covered for military veterans.[9] Hormones and mental health therapy have been provided for some time. Veterans are advised to watch for details in this very recent development.

> To transgender Americans across the country—especially the young people who are so brave—I want you to know your President has your back.
>
> During Pride Month—and all the time.
>
> — *President Biden, @POTUS, 4:31 PM, June 7, 2021*

---

[7] FSA Store, "Transgender Counseling or Surgery: FSA Eligibility," accessed July 28, 2021, https://fsastore.com/FSA-Eligibility-List/T/Transgender-Counseling-or-Surgery-E717.aspx.

[8] Dr. Christine McGinn, email message to the author, September 29, 2019.

[9] Meryl Kornfield, "VA Plans to Offer Gender-Confirmation Surgery to Transgender Veterans, Reversing Ban," *The Washington Post*, June 19, 2021, https://www.washingtonpost.com/national-security/2021/06/19/veterans-gender-affirmation-surgery/.

- **Some surgeons offer a significant discount for clients who pay cash.**
  One practice offers a 65 percent cash discount on surgical fees. Ask in advance.

- **Family members may help.**
  For some, this option will be clearly out of reach. But think about your parents and grandparents; they *may* be delighted to help you with your expenses. They may be gracious enough to gift you the funds, but never *assume* they will. Structure any funding as a *loan* that you pay back at fair terms. If you are young enough to be covered by your parents' insurance (usually up to but not including age 26), use it. Expect to do the footwork to find out what's provided.

- **Run a GoFundMe campaign to raise money for your expenses.**
  GoFundMe is a trans-supportive organization that provides an Internet platform for all kinds of fundraising. (GoFundMe has raised a collective $5 billion for various causes over their 8 years in operation, including $27 million within 30 days sent directly to folks impacted by Hurricane Harvey.) You can tell your story internationally and raise money from people who earnestly want you to meet your goal.

  There's no fee to list your plea on a GoFundMe platform and it is simple to set up. Beyond that, GoFundMe takes 2.9 percent of each donation in addition to a 30-cent fee per credit or debit transaction. *You keep the rest of the funds raised.* (On Kickstarter, conversely, you state a dollar goal but keep nothing if you don't make the goal. On GoFundMe, you keep whatever you raise, minus the fees.) You'll find a helpful blog post titled "The Ultimate Fundraising Guide for Gender Confirmation Surgery" at gofundme.com/c/blog/gender-confirmation-surgery.

- **Apply for a grant from one of these three organizations:**
  The **Jim Collins Foundation** (jimcollinsfoundation.org) provides financial assistance to fund gender-affirming surgeries for qualified applicants. Tony Ferraiolo and Dru LeVasseur started the foundation in 2008 in honor of Jim Collins, who was a licensed clinical social worker and clinical instructor in the department of psychiatry at the Yale School of Medicine. According to the Foundation website, Jim was "an avid supporter and ally to the transgender community, advocating for the right of all people to live their lives with honesty and passion." The foundation receives funds from thousands of individual donors and has been fortunate to use the pro bono services of Drs. Marci Bowers, Christine McGinn, and E. Antonio Mangubat. Applicants must be 18 years of age by the end of the foundation's annual grant cycle. Complete an application online.

  Point of Pride (pointofpride.org) is an outgrowth of Point 5cc, a clothing and accessory company that contributes 20 percent of its proceeds to provide funding assistance to trans and nonbinary people needing surgery. In 2016, Point of Pride branched off from the parent organization, becoming its own 501 (c)(3) nonprofit organization. It offers the following programs: their Annual Transgender Surgery Fund, a free chest binder program, a free trans femme shapewear program, and an electrolysis support program. Point of Pride has served thousands of trans folks in all 50 states and over 50 countries in meaningful, life-changing ways.

  Genderbands (genderbands.org) is a Utah-based nonprofit founded in 2015 to pay for the founder's top surgery. Now the organization funds gender-related surgeries for others. Genderbands receives sponsorships from several surgeons performing transgender care, sells merchandise, and offers support and social groups for the trans and gender-nonconforming community.

- **Raise money by selling things you don't need.**

Many online services allow you to sell your unneeded things for cash. Investigate OfferUp, letgo, eBay, Facebook Marketplace, thredUP, and Poshmark for selling good used clothing, or Craigslist. Maybe you have an old musical instrument or a car that would bring in some money. Sports trading cards, autographs, and other collectibles may mean less to you now that you're considering gender-affirming surgery. Even old furniture and clothing add up. You take a photo of the item you're selling, write a description, and set a price. Obviously, take *extreme* care if you are having people you don't know come to your home!

- **Get a part-time job.**
  Just when life is complicated enough, do you have time and a vehicle to allow you to drive for Uber or Lyft? Could you add a less-demanding part-time job to bring in some extra cash? Some part-time positions (such as Starbucks) offer health benefits that may cover your surgery.

- **Consider a personal loan.**
  Consider this option only with great caution. Be even more careful if you consider using a credit card. These ideas may lead you into financial hell, meaning poor credit or even bankruptcy. So, be certain about your choices here. Talk to someone you trust, such as a financial advisor who doesn't stand to profit through your decisions.

- **Consider a home equity loan if you have property.**
  Be extremely cautious if you consider this option. A home equity loan or home equity line of credit can be very risky territory. A default on this loan could result in the loss of your home.

- **Use CareCredit.**
  Our office and a variety of surgeons' offices offer CareCredit. This company allows qualified individuals to borrow money for medical procedures. Just be sure you pay it back *quickly*, or the interest rate accelerates over time, increasing the total that you owe.

Choosing Your Surgeon

Choosing a surgeon who is a good match for you is critical. It goes without saying that your surgeon must be competent—preferably excellent. But you want someone who communicates well with you, too. How do you judge? Here are some pointers.

- **Ask your own friends, healthcare provider, or therapist for some names to get you started.**

- **Look up surgeons' names and contact information through WPATH.**
  Then visit their websites and see how they present their services (wpath.org). Or in Seattle, check Ingersoll Gender Center's site (ingersollgendercenter.org).

- **Ask trans friends and contacts for information on their surgical experiences.**
  Many individuals may be willing to tell you about their experiences or even show you their results. (Of course, we are talking about consenting adults here.) Online contacts through Reddit and through monitored, invitational trans sites may also be helpful to you. Look up transgender surgeries on YouTube and Instagram as well.

- **Go to conferences; many surgeons attend national and regional transgender conferences.**
  Check out the Philadelphia Trans Wellness Conference held every summer, Gender Odyssey (originally in Seattle, but in San Diego starting in 2019), Gender Spectrum in Oakland, First Event in

Boston, Keystone in Pennsylvania, Esprit in the Pacific Northwest, and regional events held by the UCSF Transgender Center of Excellence or by WPATH (wpath.org).[10]

At these conferences, you may have the opportunity to hear a surgeon speak, see slides of their work, and ask them questions directly. Sometimes, they will even arrange an informal consultation with you. This will give you an idea of the surgeon's personality, their willingness to answer questions, and how you feel about them. (A surgeon doesn't have to be your buddy, but you should have a sense that they are sincere and have your best interests at heart. If your gut says, "I can't work with this surgeon," don't.) If you cannot attend these conferences, browse the conference websites to see which surgeons have served as financial sponsors of the event. That's not necessarily a cause for an endorsement, but it's another clue.

- **Read online reviews of different physicians.**
  Keep in mind that all physicians get "Yelped" from time to time and reviewers aren't always kind or fair. A reviewer may blast a doctor without the benefit of knowing or explaining the whole story. I've seen some vicious reviews written about outstanding surgeons.

> Ask the surgeons you're researching or their surgical coordinator if they can put you in touch with one or more of their former patients who would be willing to share their experiences with you.

- **Verify that your surgeon is board-certified.**
  In general, surgeons have completed medical school (generally for 4 years after graduating from college) and a residency (an additional 4 to 10-plus years of surgical training). They may have done a specialized fellowship for a year or longer in addition to that. The American Board of Medical Specialties certifies physicians through their inclusion requirements, CME (continuing medical education) requirements, and periodic recertification examinations. A surgeon may approach sexual reassignment surgery from a variety of disciplines: gynecology, urology, plastic surgery, and others. We are now beginning to see fellowships in transgender surgery, such as the Mount Sinai Program in New York City.

- **Research completely.**
  While board certification is a good place to start in your search, go a little further. Ask about your surgeon's education, training, and experience in the procedure you want to have. Ask how long they have been offering the procedure and how many they have performed. A surgeon may be board-certified, but if they perform a specific surgery only occasionally, you may want to continue your search until you are comfortable that your surgeon will deliver the results you want. As stated, we are beginning to see fellowships in transgender medicine and surgery, but it's still early. (At my alma mater, the University of Washington School of Medicine, transgender medicine is still offered as an elective course.)

- **Be aware that volume and experience can make a difference in quality.**

---

10 Gender Spectrum holds an annual gender conference each July that is particularly popular among trans youth and families. It has grown annually and now attracts hundreds.

Expanding on the point above, research in other surgeries (such as coronary artery bypass grafts, bariatric surgeries, and breast cancer surgeries) has established that surgical volume correlates with better outcomes.[11] According to Dr. Richard Santucci, the Crane Center reported performing a total of 108 phalloplasties and 140 vaginoplasties in 2018 alone. Not a single patient had to go back for a vascular emergency. This is impressive, considering that some centers may do only a few phalloplasties per year.

- **Find a surgeon who knows and works with the trans community.**
Make sure the surgeon knows the community, uses appropriate vocabulary, and doesn't ask unnecessarily prying questions. Try to make sure your surgeon understands the many issues that trans people encounter. You may learn this by talking to former patients, reading reviews, or getting a "gut sense" when you hear them speak.

> I had a trans male patient who needed a urologic consultation for recurrent urinary tract infections. The patient had had a metoidioplasty but not a urethral extension. He, therefore, didn't pee through the phallus—but rather through his urethra just underneath it. It was certainly appropriate that the urologist sort out the revised anatomy, but my patient was devastated when the urologist asked, "So, you mean the penis is just for show then?"
>
> I'm certain this remark was not intended to injure the patient, but it may have reflected a lack of trans competence. Fortunately, the patient was able to process the remark as a lack of sensitivity on the part of the physician rather than reflective of some personal inadequacy of his own.
>
> — Linda Gromko, MD

- **Check with the surgeon's department of medical licensing.**
A doctor must be licensed in the state in which they practice. Be certain that the surgeon's license is current and that there haven't been disciplinary actions taken or pending. Even this may not be a deal breaker, but wouldn't you want to know if your surgeon's license had been suspended?

- **Research and understand the potential complications associated with the surgery you are planning.**
Some surgeons are very open and willing to share their own complication rates for specific surgeries. (If the surgeon says they have had no complications, that's your clue to find a different surgeon.) No surgery is without risk. So, how does a surgeon manage complications that do arise? Many surgeons give patients their personal contact information, like a cell phone number, to use during the postoperative period, or they provide the number for an on-call physician.

- **Make a list of pluses and minuses about that surgeon and their approach after you've met with them and had a face-to-face consultation.**

---

11   Johannes Morche, Tim Mathes, and Dawid Pieper, "Relationship between Surgeon Volume and Outcomes: A Systematic Review of Systematic Reviews," *Systematic Reviews* 5, no. 1 (November 2016): 1, https://doi.org/10.1186/s13643-016-0376-4.

But then, give your heart a vote. How did you feel about this person? How did you feel about the staff? Were there nonverbal messages, like being treated rudely, being put on hold forever, or having your paperwork lost? All of these experiences reflect on the surgeon who sets the tone for the culture in the office. Were they trans-friendly and trans-sensitive? Most importantly, would you want your parent, spouse, or child to be in their care?

Getting Your Presurgery Letters

If you are arranging a gender-affirming surgery, your health insurance company and your surgeon will require letters of support from one or more healthcare professionals. These letters ensure that a candidate for surgery (patient) meets the Standards of Care as set forth by the World Professional Association for Transgender Health (WPATH). WPATH is a nonprofit, interdisciplinary professional and educational organization devoted to the health of transgender and gender-diverse persons. The most recent Standards of Care (SOC-8) were released on July 15, 2022. Download the new Standards of Care (SOC-8) free at **WPATH.org/publications/soc**.

You will find that WPATH Standards are offered as "recommendations" rather than firm requirements. Health insurance companies tend to accept the WPATH Standards of Care, however, and require letters based on these standards. Letter requirements vary among health insurance companies and surgeons.

Practical Pointers to Help You Get Your Letters

- Specific health insurance providers—and specific surgeons—will have their own letter requirements. Know what these requirements are *in your situation*, so you will not face last-minute barriers.

- Genital surgeries tend to require more letters from providers than do breast modifications, facial surgeries, or body contouring. When two letters are required, one letter is to be from a mental health therapist of master's level training. Another may be required from a mental health provider at the MD or PhD level (i.e., a psychiatrist or psychologist).

- Letters must be current, i.e., within one year of the surgical date. If not, your surgeon will require a more up-to-date letter.

- A letter from your hormone prescriber may be required by surgeons and insurance companies. Unless your hormone prescriber is very experienced in writing such letters, you cannot expect them to know what is required. Here is a template that may help: **transline.zendesk.com/hc/en-us/articles/229372788-Surgery-Sample-Letter**.

- More letters will be required for adolescent candidates, as will parental consent (see SOC-8, Statement 13.7).

- More letters will be required for candidates seeking individually customized or "nonstandard" surgeries (see SOC-8, Statement 13.8).

The WPATH Standards of Care ensure that a surgical candidate (patient) is likely to have a positive outcome from a requested surgery. Refer to Appendix D in SOC-8. The Standards also delineate the credentials of the surgeon, ensuring that the surgeon is qualified to perform gender-affirming surgeries. The Standards protect both surgeons and patients. (Refer to WPATH SOC-8, Statement 13.1 for surgeons' credentials.)

Facial surgery is now designated by WPATH as a gender-affirming surgical procedure (see Appendix E in WPATH SOC-8), as are many other surgeries that were not previously covered by insurance. If facial surgery is being done to manage gender dysphoria, the diagnosis must be supported. For a thorough account of the literature surrounding the medical necessity of facial surgery for trans women, see the Transgender Legal Defense and Education Fund's review.[12]

If you do not have a mental health therapist now, this is a good time to find a therapist who will write a letter in support of your having gender-affirming surgery. And since you are about to have a major life event, it might not hurt to have a therapist waiting in the wings. Google "mental health therapists who work with transgender people" in your area.

The Critical 6 Weeks Prior to Surgery

A multitude of things must be clarified, arranged, and purchased before your surgery. Hopefully, you will have a chance to read this chapter before the last minute. Use this as a checklist if it helps.

Confirm Logistical Arrangements with Your Surgeon's Office

- ❏ Double-check the date and time of your surgery.
- ❏ Confirm your arrival time at the surgical facility. Record the facility's address and phone number.
- ❏ Most surgeons require a preoperative visit to go over detailed post-op instructions, write prescriptions needed after surgery (medications for pain and nausea, and typically an antibiotic to prevent infection). Some may show you the post-op dressings and how to use them.
- ❏ Confirm that payment arrangements and insurance billing are in order.
- ❏ Find out how long you are expected to stay in the hospital or if the surgery is considered an "outpatient" or a "day surgery" where you go home on the same day of the operation.
- ❏ If you are traveling out of town for surgery, confirm the length of time the surgeon requires you to stay in town after your surgery for follow-up care.
- ❏ Confirm whether your surgeon has arrangements with an inn, local recovery house, or hotel where you will stay during your convalescence.
    - ❏ If you are to be supervised by someone during your stay at a hotel or inn, find out if the person caring for you has medical or nursing credentials. (Just know what to expect.)

---

[12] Transgender Legal Defense and Education Fund, *Medical Necessity of Facial Gender Reassignment Surgery for Transgender Women: Literature Review*, Washington, DC: Transgender Legal Defense and Education Fund, September 10, 2020, https://transhealthproject.org/documents/34/Facial_surgery_medical_necessity_literature_review.pdf.

- ❑ Remember also that you must be medically stable enough to go to an inn or hotel. Do not cut corners on your early postoperative recovery or allow someone else to suggest that you do.

- ❑ Surgeons often say that undergoing surgery is not the difficult part; recovery is. Don't risk jeopardizing your results.

❑ If you are staying out of town, find out if you yourself must arrange for a recovery facility or care providers outside the hospital.

❑ Record the name, phone number, and email address for your surgeon's contact person, which is who you'll contact if you have routine questions or concerns before or after surgery.

❑ Learn how to access the surgeon or their on-call person in an urgent situation. What is their emergency contact phone number and who will you be reaching?

Confirm Medical Arrangements with Your Surgeon's Office

❑ Ask the office staff if you need special tests from your primary care provider prior to surgery (such as an EKG, blood tests, and an HIV test).

❑ Ask if you will need a preoperative physical exam by your primary care provider. (Is there a form provided for that? How close to the day of surgery should it be completed? Or, how far in advance of the surgery may it be done?)

❑ Ask when you are supposed to stop medications prior to surgery and clarify which medications you are supposed to stop.

> It is a universal rule to not take aspirin for 10 days prior to surgery. Aspirin impairs your platelet function and can impair your blood clotting ability. NSAIDs (nonsteroidal anti-inflammatories like ibuprofen or naproxen sodium) must also be stopped ahead of time, as must vitamin E supplements.

❑ Check with your surgeon's office regarding hormones. Many surgeons will specify no hormones for 2 weeks prior to surgery, but others do not. Know your surgeon's recommendations.

❑ Ask when you can have your last electrolysis appointment prior to surgery. (About 2 to 4 weeks is common, but check with the surgeon's office.)

❑ Find out what equipment and supplies you will need to buy ahead of time, such as sanitary protection for trans male and trans female surgery or sterile lubricant for dilation (vaginal dilators are provided by the surgeon).

❑ Learn the specifics of bowel prep prior to surgery. (This is a regimen of laxatives to clean out the bowel, common in any abdominal or genitourinary surgery.)

❑ Find out if there a cancellation list so you may have your surgery earlier if someone else cancels.

- ❏ Ask if there is anything you can do to prepare yourself and your living space for recovery (see Chapter 5).

- ❏ Ask if your surgeon recommends making post-op arrangements for pelvic floor physical therapy. This modality helps people with urinary, bowel, and sexual function after gender-affirming surgery. Ask for a referral.

Dr. Bowers's Recommendations on Stopping Hormones before Surgery

For years, it was considered gospel that all patients undergoing gender-affirming surgeries would stop HRT 6 weeks before surgery. In general, they arrived miserable and basically in menopause or with recurrence of androgenic symptoms. This was never questioned until more contemporary surgeons challenged this notion as lacking evidence and allowed patients to drop to a baseline level of hormone replacement therapy, usually 6 weeks prior to surgery, and proceed with some intraoperative preventative measures such as pneumatic compression devices (sequential compression devices) and low-molecular-weight heparin (Lovanox). Patients were considerably happier and rates of thromboembolism were unaltered.

— *Marci Bowers, MD*

Note: Follow your own surgeon's advice, of course, but Dr. Bowers's comments may stimulate discussion. Madeline Deutsch, MD, of the University of California-San Francisco, echoed Dr. Bowers' comments in her presentation, "Should Estrogen Be Discontinued Prior to Surgery?," presented at the WPATH 26th Scientific Symposium Surgeon's Program on November 6, 2020.

In a review of available literature on the subject, Deutsch concluded that was no scientific evidence to support routinely stopping estradiol before surgery. (She clarified that ethinyl estradiol commonly used in birth control pills does have a higher rate of blood clotting events.)

- ❏ Ask if there are written post-op instruction sheets that you can read ahead of time. (It really does matter that you follow them. Surgery is a partnership between you, your family, your primary care providers, your surgeon, and the surgical team. Everybody must do their part to keep you safe and comfortable, and to allow you to achieve the best results possible.)

- ❏ Make a list of your medications to take with you. Note the dose of your medication, the dosing schedule (how often you are supposed to take the medicine), and know why you are taking your medications. (Know this information in advance; your providers cannot know what your "little yellow pill" is.) Some people photograph their medication labels. It doesn't matter how you do this, but take the information with you.

- ❏ Most importantly, make a list of allergies and medications you are allergic to so you can inform your medical staff.

❏ Get a copy of your EKG to take with you if you happen to have a known heart problem and your primary care provider has taken an EKG. (An old EKG is golden if you have cardiac or respiratory symptoms; comparing the old EKG with a current one provides extremely useful information.)

For facial surgery, hair removal must be stopped 1 month before surgery and cannot be started for 3 months after facial surgery. With the very few infections we've ever had in head and neck surgery (and with maybe one exception), all the patients had electrolysis or laser hair removal within a few months of surgery. Pseudomonas and other bacteria that seem to peacefully coexist within hair follicles don't bode very well if they escape by manipulating the follicle and seeding the circulatory system (during electrolysis, it is possible for bacteria in the skin or hair follicles to move into the bloodstream and cause serious infections).

— *Jordan Deschamps-Braly, MD*

Confirm Your Travel Arrangements

❏ Confirm your hotel or Airbnb reservations.

❏ Confirm airline, bus, and train tickets for you and your travel partner.

❏ Update immunizations (refer to page 12 in Chapter 1).

❏ Confirm that you have your travel documents, such as a driver's license, a US passport, or other appropriate documents for international travel.

❏ Obtain a "carry letter" if you need one. If you are carrying injectable medications, needles, and syringes, you are advised to get a carry letter from your primary care physician. (I write these on my prescription pad or office stationery, stating that "John Doe is my medical patient and requires injected hormones to treat a medical condition. Therefore, the patient is required to carry the medication, and needles and syringes for administration during travel.")

Confirm Work Arrangements

❏ Have you notified your direct supervisor and your human resources department that you will be gone? It's important to consider what information you are giving and to whom; you can be discreet about personal information. Does your company require a note from your healthcare provider? Is a note required for you to return to work?

❏ Do you need to arrange for Family and Medical Leave Act (FMLA) paperwork? The FMLA may apply to you if your company employs at least 50 people and you have worked there for 12 months (see dol.gov/general/topic/benefits-leave/fmla). FMLA applies to workers in the private sector (provided that the above conditions are met), the government or public sector, or in public or private primary or secondary schools, regardless of the number of workers. FMLA allows you to be away from work due to illness, injury, or surgery—in you or a family member—for up to 12 work weeks. *The FMLA does not provide for pay, but it does ensure that you will have your prior job or a comparable one on your return.* If you have a travel partner who qualifies for FMLA to care for you, they may apply for FMLA at their workplace also.

Your primary care physician (or your surgeon) is often the one who completes the paperwork. In my office, I do this with the patient sitting right there so there's no question how the absence is represented.

- ❏ Have you confirmed with your employer whether you qualify for sick leave or personal time off, or possibly short-term disability if it is provided by your company? If there is short-term disability, know that it comes with its own raft of paperwork. Don't be caught short because you didn't know.

Being Discreet

Be alert that if you are not "out" with respect to gender issues, your human resources department or supervisor could out you. While I'm not a proponent of lying, your privacy is critical. Here are some examples that have worked for patients of mine when they were asked for specifics:

"I'm having some female surgery." You may find that your supervisor will become embarrassed and look away. Of course, it isn't their business. And you do not have to give them specifics.

"This is quite private, but I'm having a birth defect corrected. I'd appreciate your being discreet about this." Again, it's not their business. If they feel compelled to ask for details, respond, "Like I said, its private. I really can't discuss it further." Or, "This is a painful matter for me to discuss." Say nothing more.

If you are having facial surgery, you won't be able to hide this during your recovery or when you return to work. If you're in a trans-friendly workplace, consider telling a few of your allies what's going on; you don't want to be the target of gossip when you return.

One of my patients was arranging return-to-work details with her employer, a large software company. She was very concerned about having to perform vaginal dilation three to four times per day—but her workplace was trans-friendly and did know the details of her upcoming absence.

So, she asked if her company might provide a quiet room with a recliner and a locked door for the purpose of dilating at work, but in private. The company was happy to oblige. After all, nursing mothers frequently have a private place to pump their breasts after they give birth.

— *Linda Gromko, MD*

Other Preoperative Considerations

Most of the people I treat are very excited before their surgeries; many are anxious. I think any range of emotions would be completely normal before a gender-affirmation surgery. Allow yourself some time and room for whatever emotional reaction you have.

It is important to think about your own postoperative care well in advance. If you are having a genital surgery where people won't be able to see what you've had done, you would likely get more sympathy and unsolicited support with a cast on your leg! We'll discuss all this in more detail in Chapter 5.

A temporary disabled parking permit may help streamline your postoperative recovery, particularly if you're having a more extensive surgery. You may not need one, but if you do, you'll be grateful you thought of this ahead of time. Download the form for your state's permit and take it to your doctor. (For Washington State, go to dol.wa.gov/vehicleregistration/parkingtemp.html.)

Your healthcare provider will sign this and give you a prescription indicating the diagnosis prompting the need for the parking permit, such as "Needs disability parking placard for postsurgical recovery."

— Linda Gromko, MD

Before you have your surgery, consider the following:

- ❏ Try to get your living space cleaned and organized before you leave; you're starting a new chapter. Change the sheets; wash your towels. Having some control at home can help you move through the disruption easier should you experience that.

- ❏ Buy frozen foods, pantry items, and nutritional snacks in advance—things you can keep in the refrigerator or freezer for when you get home. Know that you need extra protein to heal wounds, even surgically created ones. Think chicken, beef, pork, eggs, protein bars, peanut butter and other nut butters, and Greek yogurt. (Refer to "Postoperative Nutrition" in Chapter 5.)

- ❏ Be prepared in advance with the postoperative supplies. For vaginoplasty, they include sterile lubricant and sanitary protection. For phalloplasty, it's sanitary protection (look at "Guards" in the male sanitary protection aisle, although you may want to have some women's sanitary pads on hand, as the size of the neophallus may be too large for a conventional pad). I have had patients who appreciated having a pack of Depends (disposable incontinence underpants) at home.

- ❏ Have personal care supplies on hand in advance: clean towels and washcloths, baby wipes for cleaning, facial towelettes—anything to make you feel more comfortable.

- ❏ Think ahead about easy clothing to wear. No fancy underwear (you will leak).

- ❏ Buy a pair of knee-high compression hose to wear during flights or long periods of immobility. These prevent swelling and may prevent DVT (blood clot) formation.

- ❏ Look online for a peri bottle if you are having vaginoplasty. This is a plastic bottle with a special nozzle that you fill with warm water to rinse your perineum from front to back. The nozzle is to direct the flow of warm water, not to insert into the neovagina. (Check with your surgeon, of course.)

- ❏ Have perineal ice packs with machine-washable cloth enclosures on hand to provide postvaginoplasty relief (check online).

- ❏ Buy a curved neck pillow to sit on (the kind you find in airport kiosks) if you are having vaginoplasty. This can help keep pressure off the perineum when you're healing. (Some people do find these pillows to be aggravating; don't use one if it bothers you.)

- ❏ Buy a NutriBullet, Vitamix, or other blender that can crush ice cubes, no matter what surgery you're having. This will help you in making high-protein smoothies.

Helping Others Help You

If you are fortunate enough to have a supportive group of people who wants to check on your progress, consider designating a point person for communication. You may not want to handle a barrage of phone calls or texts; your point person can do that. Use a password-protected communication system, like the ones below:

- **Caring Bridge can help you update concerned friends (caringbridge.org).**
  This service enables people to post details about someone dealing with a surgery or illness. All concerned individuals may simply log onto the site with their password. Plus, they can make encouraging comments to support you.

- **Lotsa Helping Hands can help you organize.**
  You may find yourself in the enviable situation of having people who want to help you but don't know how to help you most effectively. If you anticipate needing extended support for meals, rides to appointments, grocery runs, and so on, look at lotsahelpinghands.com/about-us. This service allows you or your point person to set up a temporary website in advance to help you coordinate the help that you might need.

Shopping Lists for Surgery

You won't need all of the following, but review this list as you make your own plans.

- ❏ Protein-rich foods (turkey, chicken, beef, tuna, shellfish, peanut butter, cheese, cottage cheese, string cheese, Greek yogurt, eggs, protein bars). If you are a vegan, search online for "high-protein vegan foods" and you'll find plenty of options.
- ❏ High-fiber foods like fruits, vegetables, and bran muffins help to reduce or prevent constipation.
- ❏ Frozen and pantry meals
- ❏ Protein powder for smoothies
- ❏ A blender that can handle ice cubes (NutriBullet, Vitamix, etc.) for making protein smoothies
- ❏ A "grabber" device that allows you to reach items without getting up and moving around (amazon.com/grabber/s?k=grabber)
- ❏ Phone chargers with longer-than-usual cords
- ❏ Compression travel stockings from a travel store or airport kiosk
- ❏ A fever thermometer
- ❏ A neck pillow or other travel pillow to sit on
- ❏ A peri bottle for rinsing front to back (get approval from your surgeon first)
- ❏ Extra washcloths and baby wipes
- ❏ Chux pads (also called "incontinence pads," "under pads," or "puppy training pads")
- ❏ Tucks pads for hemorrhoidal care (soothing witch hazel pads for your perineum)
- ❏ Sanitary pads
- ❏ Depend Guards for Men, Depends, or sanitary pads after phalloplasty
- ❏ Sanitary pads and panty liners after vaginoplasty
- ❏ Sterile lubricant (water-based sterile lubricants like Surgilube, Slippery Stuff, or McKesson)
- ❏ Perineal ice packs (look online)
- ❏ Medical and dressing supplies: A comprehensive list of supplies is outlined on the following blog post designed for postphalloplasty care. Many of the supplies listed are appropriate for postvaginoplasty care as well. The list will familiarize you with the various products, and you won't need all of them, but it may help you organize: myphalloplasty.wordpress.com/2016/09/28/medical-supplies-packing-list (and compare it with your surgeon's office list).

If you are having a radial forearm phalloplasty, your surgeon may ask you to get a protective garment from a medical supply or burn center. Ask ahead of time if they provide this.

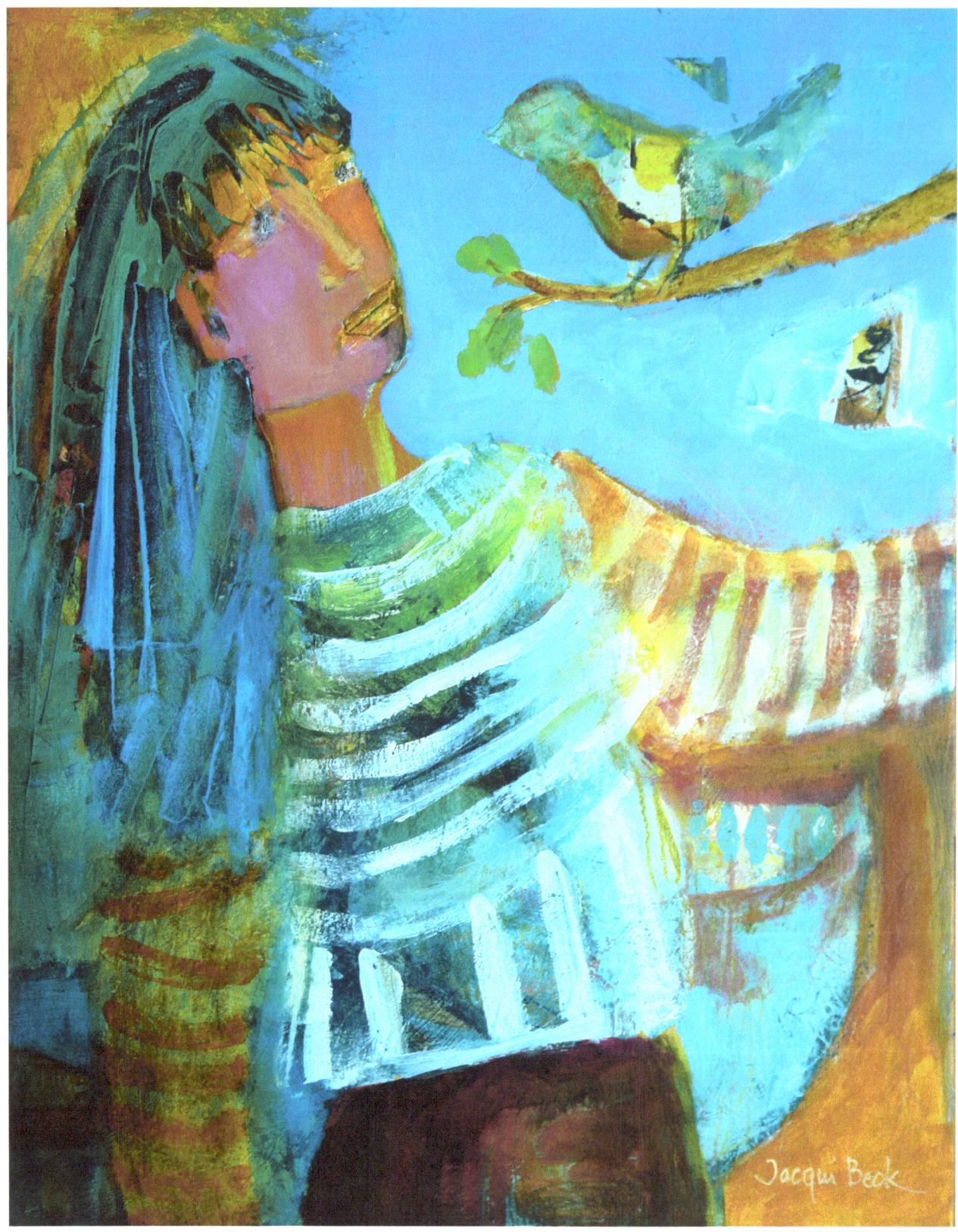

Conversation

CHAPTER 2
Feminizing Surgeries

For no specific reason, we will begin by discussing feminizing surgeries and follow with masculinizing surgeries.

Keep in mind that all surgeons do even the same surgeries slightly differently. If a surgeon has developed a style of doing a procedure, it probably means that they have found specific ways that work best for them and for their patients. *It doesn't mean that one way is right or wrong or that one doctor's approach is the only way to perform a given surgery.*

Surgeons and patients alike can be quite opinionated when it comes to styles of surgery. Just keep an open mind as you read and gather your own questions in advance to prepare yourself in the best way possible.

In this chapter, we will discuss each of the gender-affirming surgeries available (or at least most of them). In Chapters 4, 5, and 6, we'll go into emergencies, the postoperative period in general, and postoperative information for specific surgeries, respectively.

Disclaimer

The information provided here is intended to give you an overview on gender-affirming surgeries. It is not intended as medical advice for you personally.

For medical advice pertaining to you specifically, seek your answers from your surgeon and their surgical team. They are the obvious professionals who will have the answers pertaining to your body and your circumstances. Information provided by them must be given more weight than my input.

You will also note that I am not including photos of surgical outcomes. They are widely available on the websites of the surgeons.

Facial Feminization Surgery

When we think of facial feminization surgery (FFS), it is more accurate to think of FFS as a *collection* of surgeries that feminize the head and neck. Individuals may be advised to have several or all of the surgeries discussed. Changing one area of the face almost always impacts the appearance of adjacent structures and the overall proportions of the face. A surgeon experienced in gender-affirming surgeries will likely appreciate these subtleties and be able to discuss them with you.

As we begin to discuss facial feminization surgery, let's look at the common differences between the facial structure of people assigned male at birth (AMAB) and people assigned female at birth (AFAB). These are the facial features that declare "male" or "female" from across a room. Remember that most people don't work all that hard to figure out another person's gender, but they do respond to reliable, stereotypical clues.

Remember that children's faces start out essentially the same. Assigned male faces develop differently under the influence of testosterone beginning in puberty. Look at the following photos of stereotypically male and female faces, and notice the following differences (we know *nothing* about the gender identity of these models):

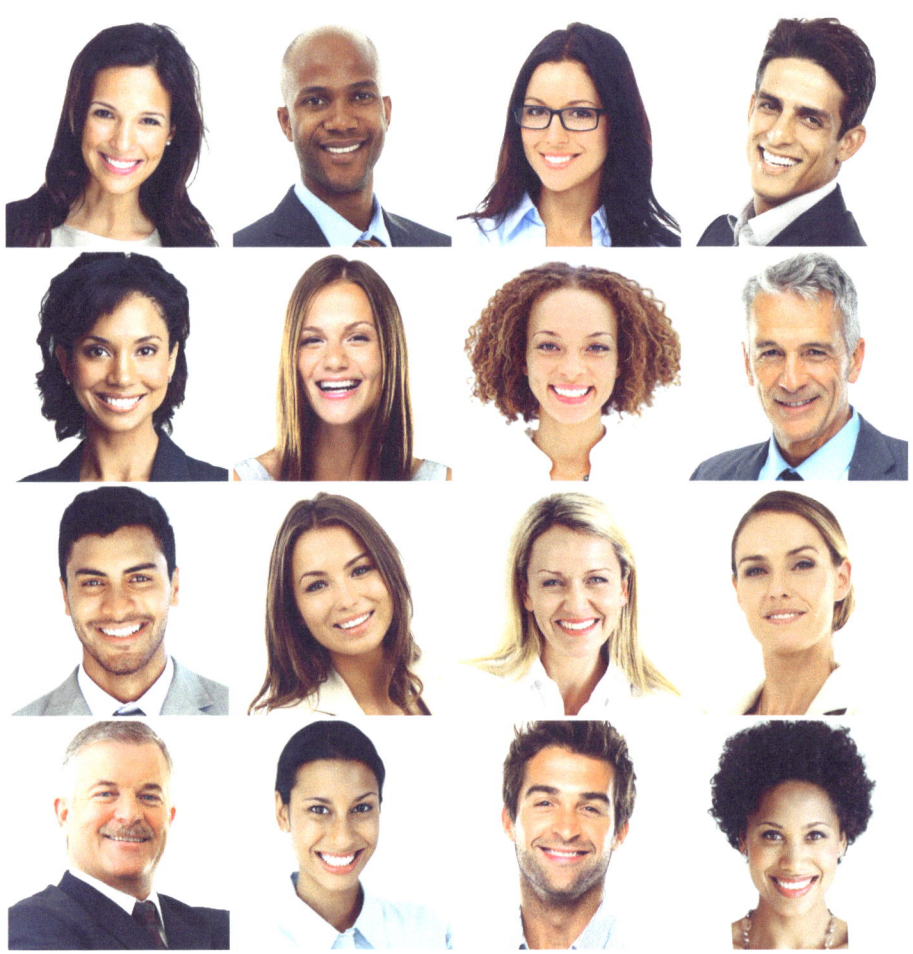

Figure 2.1. Stereotypically male and female faces.

- Brow bones—that is, the bone of the central forehead above and between the brows—tend to be more prominent in males. So are the bones over the outer brow and above the eyes.

- Brows tend to rest lower on the supraorbital ridge (the bony rim on the upper part of the eye socket) in males. In females, the brows appear higher and more arched.

- The male forehead may appear higher or longer from the brow to the hairline.

- The male hairline tends to be squarer or more peaked with less hair in the temples, while a more feminine hairline is rounder in shape.

- A receding hairline or baldness is likely to be read as male.

- Cheekbones are stereotypically less defined in males than in females. This difference is more the result of soft tissue than of bone volume. Other factors, such as racial and genetic differences, may influence cheek structure also.

- The male nose tends to be larger and longer, with males having a less defined tip and females having a slightly curved tip.

- The male upper lip tends to be longer from the bottom of the nose to the top of the lip.

- The male lips (upper and lower) are often less full than in females.

- The male jaw appears larger, broader, and more angular.

- The male chin appears longer, wider, squarer, and more forward than the female chin.

- The Adam's apple may be quite prominent in the male. The Adam's apple is made of thyroid cartilage, and both assigned males and assigned females have them. As with other changes, it is the influence of testosterone that makes the prominent Adam's apple recognizable as a male trait.

All of these are general guidelines for attractive males or females who fit within an ideal of aesthetic norms. I think it is helpful to explain that these are not absolute criteria and that a person shouldn't be compelled to change a part of their face that they like or want to preserve. Sometimes they like a feature because it is similar to that of a parent, brother, or sister.

— *Toby Meltzer, MD*

Examine these photos of the skulls of assigned males and assigned females. You'll spot the bony differences easily.

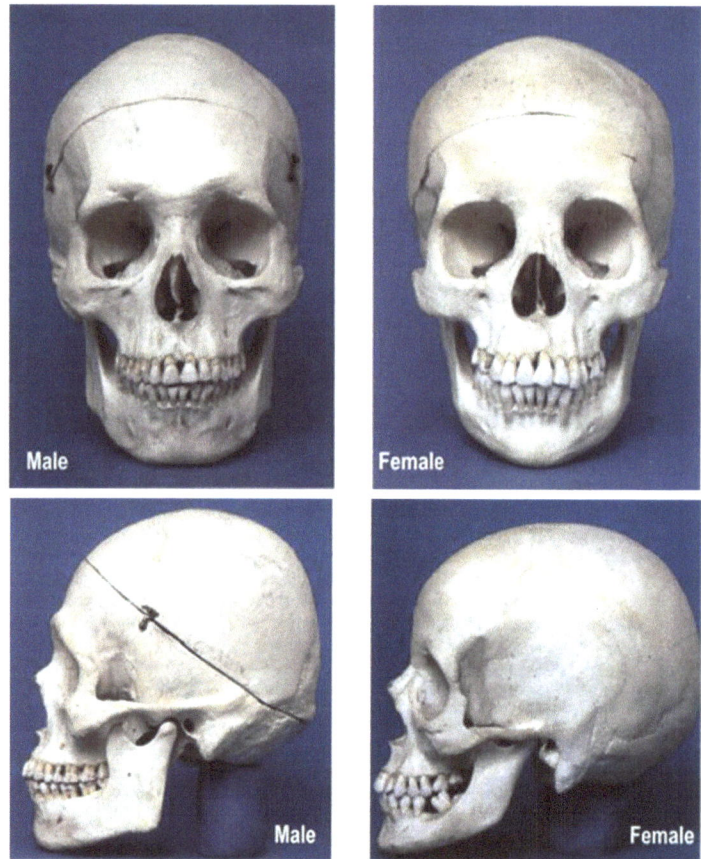

Figure 2.2. Differences in the skulls of assigned males and females.

When you consult a surgeon regarding FFS, the surgeon will examine your facial structures carefully. Images of the face, such as CT scans, CT scans with 3D reconstruction, cephalometric X-rays, or MRI scans, may be used to define your facial bones precisely. Your surgeon may ask to see photos of other females in your family. They will also ask about your personal objectives, such as what *you* want to see happen as a result of your surgery.

The surgeon will make recommendations based on your facial structure and your goals. As stated earlier, FFS is best represented as a *collection* of surgical procedures. Some women will be advised to have all of the components of FFS, while others to have relatively few. Remember that when you change one part of your face, the rest of it may appear off-balance unless other portions are changed as well. This truly calls for an expert opinion, and preferably from a surgeon who does FFS routinely.

Surgeons vary from one another in how they evaluate a face prior to surgery. For instance, the surgeons of Facialteam in Spain use CT scans with 3D reconstruction. A 3D printer can be used to create personalized cutting guides for surgery on the lower jaw. If forehead work is to be done, a 3D reconstruction from a CT scan informs the surgeon of the exact boundaries and the size of the frontal sinuses in the forehead.

FFS Is a Collection of Surgeries

In many facial feminization surgeries, you'll see the following modifications:

- **Brow bone reduction**
  The brow bone may be shaved and rounded. There are several approaches.

  - One surgeon says, "Shaving with a burr [a drill bit that cuts bone] is possible in about one-third of patients. In the remainder, the anterior wall of the forehead is removed, reshaped, and put back down. Bone over the outer brow is frequently reduced. Bone from the orbit around the eye is frequently removed to shape the eye."

  - Another surgeon comments, "Burring alone tends to be sufficient in about 2 to 3 percent of patients."

- **Scalp advance**
  This brings the hairline forward and makes the forehead appear less pronounced. An added benefit of a hairline advancement is often a brow lift that further feminizes the face.

- **Hair transplants**
  Harvested from the base of the skull, the transplants fill in areas of androgynous alopecia (male pattern hair loss), often one to three follicles at a time. Keep in mind that to gain the hair density required for a female hairline, most patients require two to three transplant procedures.

- **Brow lift**
  This elevates and shapes the eyebrows, creating a feminine arch.

- **Rhinoplasty (nose job)**
  This creates a smaller, more feminine-appearing nose. A female nose is often more delicate and upturned than a male nose; it is often narrower and more "refined."

- **Cheek implants**
  These accent the cheekbones. Implants imply that solid silicone, Gortex, or a type of hard plastic is inserted, while grafts are transfers of fat or bone from other parts of the body.

- **Lip lift**
  This reduces the distance between the lower edge of the nose and the upper lip, rotates the upper lip upward and outward, and creates a shorter, more feminine appearance. By shortening the lip, you create more dental "show," which also creates a more female appearance. Lip contouring with implants may also help to make the lips look fuller.

- **Chin and mandible contouring**
  The chin is rounded and the angles of the jaw are softened and reduced. The jaw bones are usually accessed from inside the mouth. Some surgeons make an exterior incision so it can be hidden, such as under the chin. The jaw can also be reduced with a technique called "reduction genioplasty." In this procedure, the chin may be reduced vertically in length and horizontally in projection.

- **Tracheal shave**
  The thyroid cartilage (Adam's apple) is shaved down to make it less prominent. The incision is hidden below the chin or in a neck crease. It is common to see this procedure done alone without other facial feminization procedures.

- **Facelift**
  Excess skin is removed and the lower and midface are tightened and repositioned to provide a more youthful appearance. Incision lines may be camouflaged immediately in front of and behind the ears and the hairline. A separate incision, similar to a tracheal shave incision below the chin, is used to tighten the neck. This is commonly done in middle-aged and older individuals.

- **Fat grafting**
  This adds contour or fullness to areas such as the cheeks, lips, and nasolabial folds.

Q Is it possible to do FFS on a teenager?

A It is medically possible. Dr. Daniel Simon and Dr. Luis Capitán of the Facialteam stated at the WPATH 26th Scientific Symposium Surgeon's Program in 2020 that one could perform FFS on a teenager. However, in addition to imaging the face, they would recommend performing a bone age test to confirm the closure of the growth plates.[13]

In addition to the above, we may see implants placed in the lips, the chin, and the sides of the temples—in other words, a *combination* of surgeries customized for each individual patient. The Facialteam in Spain has published a protocol that describes the sequence in which they perform FFS.[14] They begin by contouring the Adam's apple and move upward to reconfigure the lower jaw. Then they perform forehead reconstruction; next, they do rhinoplasty. They finish with the more minor aesthetic procedures, such as blepharoplasty, lip lifts, implants, or injections.

Vocal feminization surgery, specifically cricothyroid approximation and feminization laryngoplasty, which are approached through the front of the neck, can be done at the same time as the tracheal shave. Endoscopic vocal cord shortening is done through the mouth and leaves no external scar. This is done during a separate surgery that allows plenty of healing time before an endotracheal intubation is performed.

FFS isn't easy to go through, according to most of my patients who have had it. Most people experience pain, bruising, and temporary swelling. But it can make the biggest possible difference in a person's *outward* presentation.

> I cannot overemphasize the importance of not smoking. The face has a rich blood supply that promotes healing. But you will always heal better and faster if you don't smoke. Stop smoking—or using *any* tobacco products—today if this is an issue for you. Ask your healthcare provider if you need help in quitting.
>
> — *Linda Gromko, MD*

---

[13] Luis Capitán, "Management of Complex Revision Frontal Sinus and Forehead Cases," (presentation, WPATH 26th Scientific Symposium Surgeon's Program, November 6, 2020).

[14] Capitán et al, "Facial Gender Confirmation Surgery: A Protocol for Diagnosis, Surgical Planning, and Postoperative Management," *Plastic and Reconstructive Surgery* 145, no. 4 (April 2020): 818e–28e, https://doi.org/10.1097/prs.0000000000006686.

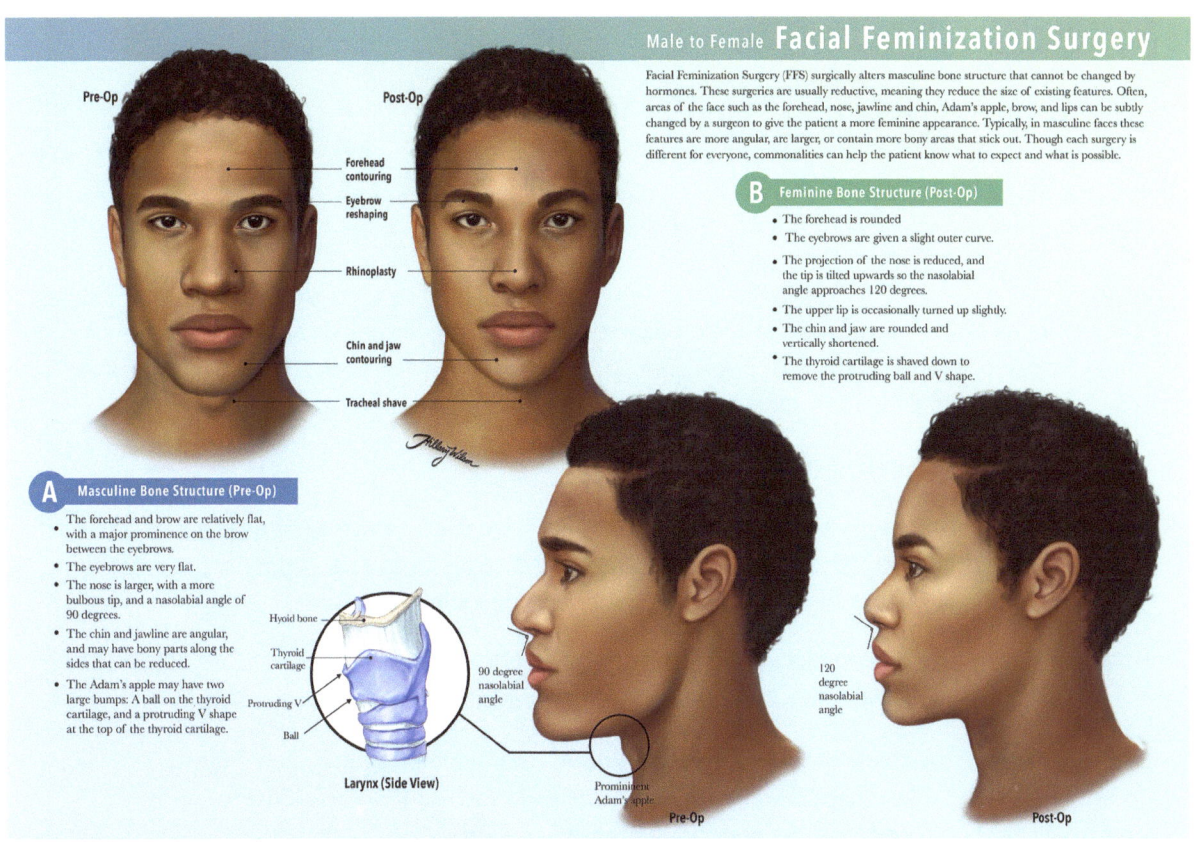
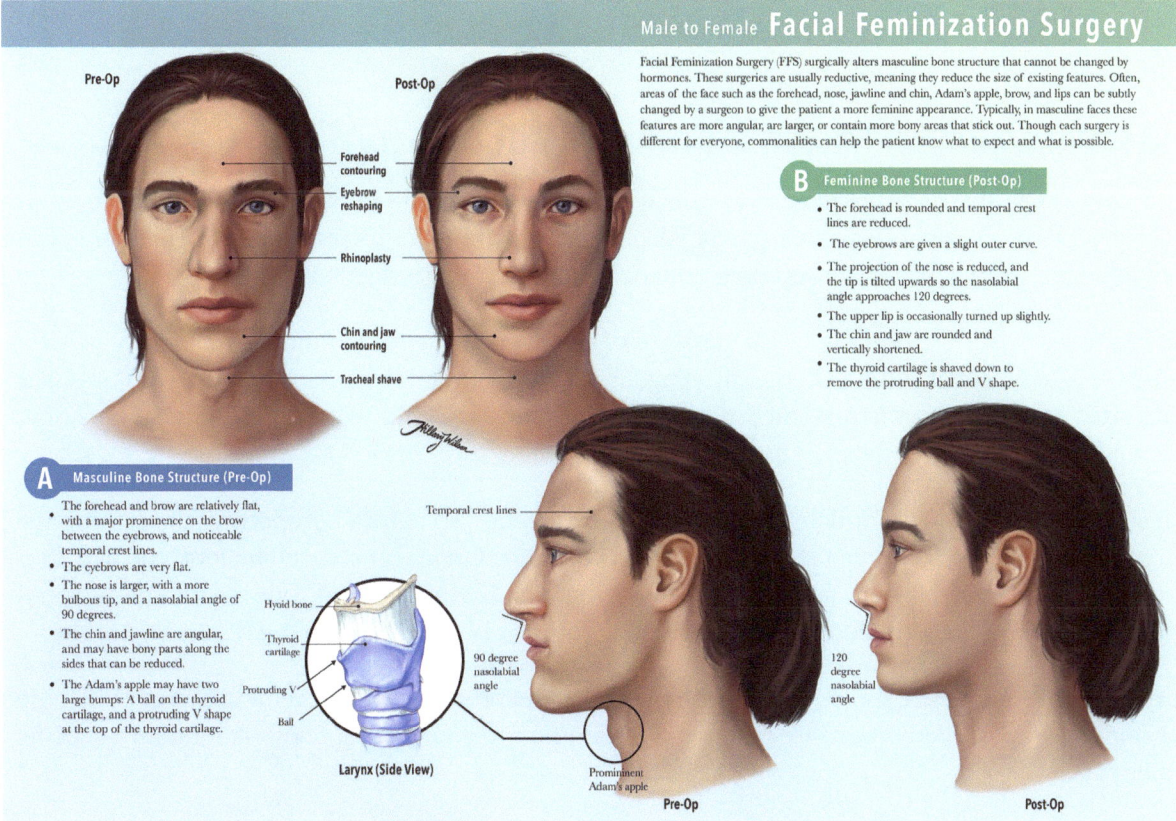

Figure 2.3. Facial feminization surgery.

Vocal Feminization Surgery and ET Tubes

Vocal feminization surgery is beyond the scope of this book. However, the following abbreviated information may be useful.

Most surgeries are done with anesthetic gas and oxygen provided by an endotracheal tube (ET tube). The ET tube is placed through the mouth, beyond the back of the throat, and between the vocal cords before it lands at the base of the mainstem bronchus where the bronchi move out to the left and right lungs. The patient, of course, is sedated with IV medication before this is done.

There are two main approaches to vocal feminization surgery:

- **The cricothyroid approximation and laryngoplasty** are done via an incision that goes through the front of the neck. This surgery tightens the vocal cords by changing their angle with respect to other structures, such as the thyroid and cricothyroid cartilage.

- **The endoscopic glottoplasty (Wendler glottoplasty)** is done via an endoscopy tube that is placed in the back of the throat; the vocal cords are sutured together to shorten them.

Intubation can occasionally damage the vocal cords. Care must be taken to allow the vocal cords to heal before any subsequent intubations. A smaller endotracheal tube or a different form of anesthesia (such as laryngeal mask anesthesia) may be needed.

Breast Enlargement (Augmentation Mammoplasty)

Breasts come in all shapes and sizes, and people have very strong opinions as to what's best for them. You will likely get most of the breast development you can expect after about 3 years on estrogen. Some women see additional growth when progesterone is added, but this is highly individual.

What implant size is best? There is a wide variation of normal breast sizes in humans. The "correct" size will depend on your vision of your desired body image. You will be given the opportunity to try on bras with various sizes of breast forms (sizers) tucked into the cups of the bra. This will help give you an idea of what size you like best.

Make sure that you wear appropriate clothing to the consultation so you can properly evaluate your new look. Wearing a sweatshirt will not show your proper contours. Once you choose the look you like, the size of the implant will be measured. Taking into account your size preference and your chest dimensions, you and your surgeon will determine the best implant size for your body to achieve the results you desire.

Implant sizes may be described in terms of volume and are expressed in cubic centimeters or cc.[15] It often helps think of your desired breast size in terms of proportion to your overall body, rather than a specific number of cc.

---

15   For reference, there are 30 cc in an ounce and 240 cc in a liquid measuring cup. In one small study, implant volumes for trans women ranged from 350 cc to 700 cc, with an average breast implant volume of 520 cc (480 cc is 1 pint).

> **Talk about your breast size preferences with your partner or a good friend who will tell you the truth. Bigger isn't always better. Large breasts are heavier and may result in soreness of your upper back and shoulders. Take your surgeon's recommendations seriously and listen to the other people whose opinions you value. But remember, the final decision about what *you* want is yours.**
>
> — *Linda Gromko, MD*

Since many trans women have broader shoulders and a wider chest than cisgender women, a trans woman may be able to accommodate a larger cup size and implant size without looking out of proportion. This is where a surgeon who is highly experienced in the subtleties of trans surgery may be a better choice than a plastic surgeon with less transgender experience.

In general, breast implants are composed of a silicone shell that is filled with either saline (basically, saltwater) or a cohesive silicone gel. Note that the latest generation of silicone implants is filled with *cohesive gel* silicone rather than liquid silicone. In the event of a rupture, cohesive silicone gel stays together, rather than leaking out into the surrounding tissues.

The implants may be placed into the chest—

- over the pectoralis muscle (one of the chest muscles) as in the drawing on the left, or
- under the pectoralis muscle as in the drawing on the right.

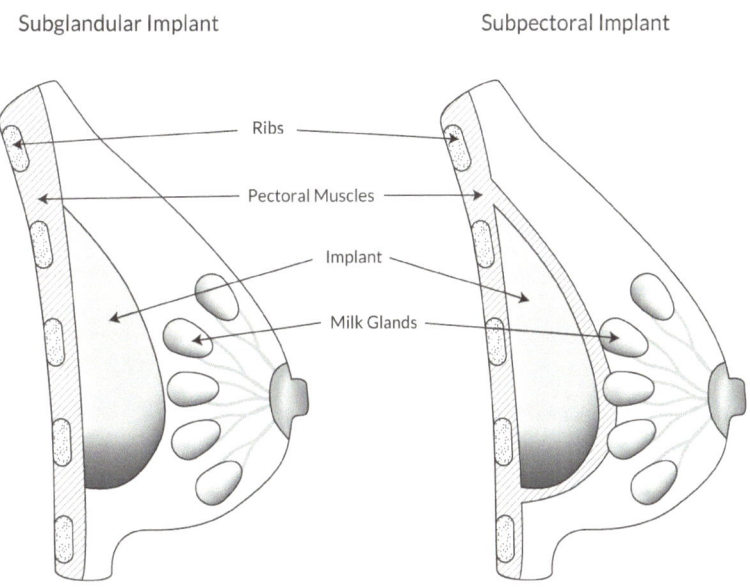

Figure 2.4. Breast implants over the pectoralis muscle (one of the chest muscles)— also called a "subglandular" implant, as in the drawing on the left—or under the pectoralis muscle, also called a "subpectoral" implant, as in the drawing on the right.

In both techniques, the implants are placed under the actual glandular tissue of the breasts. If the over-the-muscle technique is used, a woman must have enough breast tissue to camouflage the implant beneath it. Otherwise, you will see the margins of the implant and it will look unnatural. For many trans women, placing the implant under the pectoralis muscle is more favorable because it provides enough soft tissue coverage to create a smooth, natural-appearing breast. Placing the implant under the muscle may also reduce the risk of a complication called capsular contracture.

Incisions for augmentation can be placed as follows:

- In the armpit (axillary approach)
- Under the lower crease of the breast (inframammary incision)
- Along the lower margin of the areola (periareolar)
- Transumbilical breast augmentation (TUBA). This is the newest of the approaches listed. An incision is hidden in the hood of the umbilicus (belly button) and tunneled into the chest area. As of the time of this writing, this technique can be done only with saline implants because they can be inserted completely deflated and then filled with saline after proper placement. For more information, refer to an article by Dr. Richard V. Dowden, "Transumbilical Breast Augmentation Is Safe and Effective."[16]

Augmentation mammoplasty is typically performed as an outpatient surgery (also called short-stay, ambulatory, or day surgery) under general anesthesia.

The Rice Test: Determining Breast Size and Breast Implant Size

Note: Dr. Scott Mosser makes the following information available to his clients so they can explore breast implant sizing at home.

Dr. Mosser will let you try on implants during your consult. The breast implants are usually tried on underneath a sports bra or in a regular-type bra. Dr. Mosser may suggest that you try on different sizes at home using the "Rice Test." Even though it is widely known as the Rice Test, we have found many materials that work better than rice for measuring volume. Particularly good is quinoa (although it's expensive), but other options that are light and a bit better than rice are oatmeal, potato flakes, and grits.

Instructions

Fill knee-high hose (or cut-off pantyhose) with the desired amount of rice, using the cc conversions listed below. Avoid using zipper-lock bags because of their pointed corners. Once you have the hosiery filled, try on the "implants" under a sports bra or under a somewhat snug underwire bra that is sheer and has no padding at all. A sports bra is helpful, especially if you plan on having your implants placed under the muscle. The sports bra compresses the breast implant sizers much like the

---

16   Richard V. Dowden, "Transumbilical Breast Augmentation Is Safe and Effective," *Seminars in Plastic Surgery* 22, no. 1 (February 2008): 51–9, https://doi.org/10.1055/s-2007-1019143.

muscle will compress the real implants. If you are going under the muscle, you'll need to add about 15 percent more to the amount that you like.

For example, if you like the way that 400 cc looks under the sports bra, you need to add 15 percent to that amount (which equates to 460-cc implants) to achieve the look you see with the 400-cc implant sizers in the sports bra.

How to Measure for CC Amount with the Rice Test

The conversions below (from cups to cubic centimeters) are approximate and will help you when doing the Rice Test.

- 1 cup = 236 cc
- ½ cup = 118 cc
- ¾ cup = 177 cc
- ¼ cup = 59 cc
- 1/3 cup = 78 cc
- 2/3 cup = 156 cc
- 1/8 cup = 30 cc

Do *not* weigh the rice. The rice must be measured as **volume** using the system above. The measurements above can be used in different combinations to achieve the cc amount you desire. It's important to remember that you should not solely rely on cc amounts just based on the photos of other patients with different body types. For instance, if you like the way that 400 cc looks on one person, that does not mean that 400 cc will give you the same look.

This is due to several things, including—but not limited to—the amount of breast tissue, shape of the chest wall, deformities of the chest wall (such as pectus excavatum and pectus carinatum), and overall body weight, to name a few. Therefore, you should do the Rice Test to give you an idea of how many cubic centimeters you may need to get the size you want.

Please remember that the Rice Test is not an exact science and is meant only to give you a rough estimate.

Possible Complications Associated with Breast Implants

Anesthesia-related complications and allergic reactions are rare, but they can occur in the perioperative period, as with any surgery. These include allergic reactions, low blood pressure, aspiration pneumonia, and peripheral nerve damage (from spinal or epidural anesthesia).

Other potential complications include infection, malposition or migration of implants, formation of hematomas (collections of blood), or rarely, seromas (collections of clear serous fluid under the skin). Hematomas and seromas may resolve spontaneously or require draining by the surgeon.

A capsular contracture occurs when normal scar tissue around an implant begins to contract and squeeze the implant, creating a firm, unnatural feel. The exact cause of contracture formation is unknown. They occur about 10 percent of the time; 90 percent of patients have the expected soft result. Contractures are graded according to the Baker Grading Scale as follows: Grade I (perfectly soft), Grade II (firm but retaining a natural appearance), Grade III (firm and misshapen), and Grade IV (firm, misshapen, and painful). A distorted appearance often requires another surgery to repair it, increasing the risk of another contracture.[17]

> Although there is no solid evidence that any postoperative treatment can decrease capsular contracture, external massage, certain oral nutraceuticals (milk thistle and vitamin E), and the asthma medications montelukast (Singulair)[18] and zafirlukast (Accolate) have been reported to decrease contractures. It is important to understand that capsular contractures are not 100 percent avoidable and may require another surgery.
>
> — E. Antonio Mangubat, MD

Another complication is implant rupture (a tear in the outer shell of an implant). When saline implants rupture, the breast deflates completely and the breasts appear asymmetric. Modern silicone gel implants are semisolid and do not leak like the older liquid silicone implants did (liquid silicone was used before 2000). With any leak, the semisolid silicone tends to remain within the implant capsule. The condition can be confirmed by magnetic resonance imaging (MRI).

Some patients with breast implants have reported systemic (total body) symptoms such as fatigue, memory loss, rash, joint pain, and brain fog—collectively termed "breast implant illness" or BII. This poorly understood syndrome continues to invite investigation, and the FDA requests adverse event reporting should such symptoms occur (1-800-FDA-1088) or online at MedWatch (fda.gov/safety/medwatch-fda-safety-information-and-adverse-event-reporting-program).

> An important mindset to have when getting breast augmentation is that this type of surgery may require maintenance. If any of the complications above occur over the course of your life, you may require surgery to address them. Implants do not need to replaced preemptively, but they do need to be replaced if they rupture, become infected, or develop capsular contracture.
>
> — Thomas Satterwhite, MD

---

17 US Food and Drug Administration, "Risks and Complications of Breast Implants," updated September 28, 2020, https://www.fda.gov/medical-devices/breast-implants/risks-and-complications-breast-implants#Capsular_Contracture.

18 Catherine K. Huang, and Neal Handel, "Effects of Singulair (Montelukast) Treatment for Capsular Contracture," *Aesthetic Surgery Journal* 30, no. 3 (July 2010): 404–8, https://doi.org/10.1177/1090820x10374724.

> ### Breast Implant-Associated Anaplastic Large-Cell Lymphoma (BIA-ALCL)
>
> A possible association between breast implants and anaplastic large-cell lymphoma was identified by the US Food and Drug Administration in 2011. The World Health Organization designated breast implant-associated anaplastic large-cell lymphoma (BIA-ALCL) as a T-cell lymphoma that can develop following breast implants. This condition is not a breast cancer but rather a type of non-Hodgkin's lymphoma (a cancer involving the immune system).
>
> Symptoms of pain or swelling, often occurring years after implant placement, should be evaluated. BIA-ALCL has been reported with both saline and silicone gel implants, although textured surfaces of implants are thought to carry a higher risk. Implant removal, chemotherapy, and radiation treatment are used to treat BIA-ALCL. For more information, read the FDA report as well as common questions and answers at fda.gov.*
>
> * US Food and Drug Administration, "Questions and Answers about Breast Implant-Associated Anaplastic Large Cell Lymphoma (BIA-ALCL)," updated October 23, 2019, https://www.fda.gov/medical-devices/breast-implants/questions-and-answers-about-breast-implant-associated-anaplastic-large-cell-lymphoma-bia-alcl.

Body Contouring

Body contouring is basically an aesthetic procedure or a set of procedures that reduces fat from some areas and adds a contouring material (such as transferred fat, implants, or dermal filler) to other areas.

Nonsurgical Body Contouring

Available for both feminizing and masculinizing are a variety of *nonsurgical* techniques for removing fat, including CoolSculpting (cryolipolysis or freezing fat) and LaserLipo (a technique for removing fat by melting it). These techniques work on fairly small areas like an abdominal pooch or flanks.

To reduce a double chin, you may want to explore CoolSculpting or Kybella injections. Kybella consists of several injections placed directly into the fat under the chin. Kybella is deoxycholic acid, a chemical that dissolves fat when injected directly into the fat under the chin. (Don't plan your photo opportunity for the next day, however; many people experience significant under-the-chin swelling before the fat lessens.)

These procedures are generally less effective than surgical contouring in that they are best suited for smaller areas and cannot claim to have the results of the surgical techniques. That said, clients who cannot afford the downtime or expense of surgery may find them to be very acceptable alternatives.

Surgical Body Contouring

If you are looking for a more extensive body modification rather than focusing on a limited area, you will likely have better—and even less costly results—from a combination of *surgical* techniques.

Liposuction can remove unwanted fat from specific areas. That fat can be recycled by sterilely processing and reinjecting it to enhance other areas of one's own body (but there's no possibility of fat donations to other people!). This is commonly done to enhance the buttocks, face, and even the breasts. You can appreciate how this requires an artistic eye and a surgeon experienced in working with gender-variant individuals.

Tumescent liposuction is the cornerstone of surgical fat removal. Here's how it works:

1. After the patient is relaxed (by general anesthesia or IV sedation), fluid is injected into the area to be treated.

2. The injected fluid consists of a mixture of saline (sterile saltwater), lidocaine (an anesthetic), and epinephrine (adrenaline). Lidocaine reduces postoperative pain. Epinephrine constricts blood vessels, significantly decreasing blood loss and postoperative bruising, and permits time to sculpt the areas of liposuction.

3. Using a variety of techniques, the fat is liquified and suctioned out using a cannula (tube) in the planned areas of fat reduction.

4. The harvested fat is processed by separating it from the other fluid. It is then recycled by reinjecting it into another area where the patient wants more volume, or it can be discarded.

After the surgery, the patient wears a compressive support garment around-the-clock for a prescribed number of weeks. Following this period, the garment may be worn less, perhaps only at night. Patients should take some downtime—such as about a week off work—and avoid heavy lifting and strenuous activity.

A return to normal activities generally depends on a person's comfort level. One surgeon's rule-of-thumb: "You may drive your car if you do not require pain medications." Some patients require no pain meds; others medicate for 2 weeks. The average postoperative medication period is about 5 days.

Tumescent liposuction can be applied in any area with superficial fat: face, neck, "bra fat," back, arms, abdomen, waist, hips, buttocks, and the legs, including the thighs, calves, knees, and ankles. It can be used on the mons area (fat above the pubic bone). Trans men in particular may seek liposuction to remove feminine-appearing fat around the hips and buttocks. Some ask that the harvested fat be transferred to the waist to camouflage a more feminine curve or placed in the chest to augment the pectoralis muscle. And some physically fit patients request sculpting their six-pack abs.

Tumescent liposuction can be combined with skin removal following massive weight-loss procedures (such as bariatric surgeries that result in the weight loss of 100 pounds or more). Tummy tucks, body lifts, and thigh lifts are commonly requested. You may also have the opportunity to create a waistline and to spot-reduce arm fat and bra fat that really cannot be exercised away.

While the fat cells that are removed from your body are gone forever, if you gain weight, your remaining fat cells can enlarge. Your results will always be better if you exercise and maintain healthy eating.

Risks of Tumescent Liposuction

Tumescent liposuction carries risks of infection, bleeding, bruising, damage to tissues, asymmetry, and contour irregularities (lumpiness). You could have an allergic reaction to the medications used, including anesthesia and pain relievers. You won't lose cellulite, and your results may not be as flawless or as symmetrical as you had hoped. You will incur expenses that are not likely to be covered by insurance, and you'll bear the cost of an enforced time away from work, if that is a concern for you.

Doing the Math: Is an Aesthetic Procedure Worth It?

Body contouring and other aesthetic procedures may be covered by insurance at times and be considered reconstructive in the setting of gender confirmation surgery. But suppose your insurance doesn't cover it. Can you afford it? Let's do some math.

Suppose you're contemplating a surgery that costs $15,000. You are 50 years old. Your parents lived to be 85 and 95. You are generally healthy and don't smoke or participate in risky activities that could shorten your life. Let's calculate the procedural cost but spread it out over your anticipated lifespan—maybe 40 more years if you live to 90 years of age. (Of course, this does not count the potential growth of this money if used in other ways.)

Cost = $15,000 divided by (40 years) = $375 per year of your life

Cost per day of remaining life: $15,000 divided by (40 years x 365 days/year) = $1.03 per day ($2.05 per day if you lived 20 years)

Q Isn't this just a rationalization for spending a lot of money on appearance?

A Perhaps, but what is the cost of living for years with something that makes you uncomfortable every single day?

Q Doesn't this sound like something reserved for the "privileged?"

A In the past, plastic surgery was the exclusive domain of the privileged. But we are beginning to see these surgeries covered by insurance for the medical treatment of gender dysphoria.

More Body Contouring: Lifting and Filling

We have already discussed breast augmentation, which is an excellent example of filling an area that requires more volume. The breast contour is enhanced by using saline or silicone implants that are placed by way of the armpit under the breast, under the areola, or through the navel.

Here are other examples:

- **The Brazilian butt lift (BBL)**
  Estradiol helps to feminize the body shape to some extent. But if you want a fuller, rounder butt and want tissue sculpted away from the waist, flank, or abdominal area, it may be possible to have a fat transfer. Fat is removed by tumescent liposuction and injected into the buttocks in sections via a large syringe and cannula. Because the fat tissue is a person's own fat, there is no risk of an immune reaction to a foreign substance—that is, no rejection. This is a popular surgery in AMAB individuals, as their buttocks are quite flat. Additionally, one can have contouring to slim the waist, which emphasizes the butt contour even more. This combination of reduction and augmentation in the same setting has been popular and successful.

- **Butt-contouring implants**

  Silicone implants can be used to add volume to the butt. They are placed through a vertical incision in the gluteal crease (the crack in the butt) under the gluteus maximus muscle so you do not sit on them. This is particularly suited for patients with little or no fat to harvest. Getting implants, however, carries the added risks of discomfort, malposition, and infection.

- **Injections to increase volume**

  Various injectable fillers may be used to add volume. These are considered temporary and are also "off-label"—that is, not FDA-approved for enhancing butt volume.

Be an Informed Consumer

Because of a number of deaths related to fat emboli, Brazilian butt lifts are controversial and have been banned in some areas. (A fat embolus is similar to a pulmonary embolus from a blood clot, except that the blockage results from transferred fat landing within a large vein and traveling north to the heart and the blood vessels in the lungs.) This is more likely to happen if large volumes of fat are injected into muscle tissue with large blood vessels. Do check with your surgeon about complications and practices aimed at reducing fat emboli before you sign up for a larger butt.

An Important Warning about Liquid Silicone Injections*

Although we don't see this much in the Pacific Northwest, many trans women have been seriously harmed by illegal silicone injections for body contouring. I'm not talking about off-label use on an otherwise FDA-approved product but about industrial chemicals, like the silicone caulking found in hardware stores and other products like paraffin and glue that black-market "pump" doctors use to inject their "patients" (victims) in hotel rooms.

Long-term effects include disfigurement of tissue, infection, and the spread of silicone to other parts of the body, producing kidney damage, stroke, and pulmonary emboli. Free or discount-cost silicone injections to any part of the body to add volume are **not** recommended.

* US Food and Drug Administration, "FDA Warns about Illegal Use of Injectable Silicone for Body Contouring and Associated Health Risks," November 13, 2017, https://www.fda.gov/news-events/press-announcements/fda-warns-about-illegal-use-injectable-silicone-body-contouring-and-associated-health-risks.

Feminizing Genital Surgeries

Orchiectomy

Bilateral orchiectomy refers to the surgical removal of the testicles. This may be performed as a surgery separate from vaginoplasty. Orchiectomy may be requested in a woman who simply wishes to stop taking testosterone blockers, or a woman who wants a surgery that is less extensive than vaginoplasty. After a bilateral orchiectomy, a person will have a flatter-appearing scrotum but still have a penis and scrotum. (Bilateral orchiectomy is a routine part of vaginoplasty in gender-affirmation surgery.)

Orchiectomy is more commonly performed as part of the treatment of testicular or prostate cancer. When it is performed to treat gender dysphoria, WPATH standards are observed (meaning the medical standards set by the World Professional Association for Transgender Health, a nonprofit, interdisciplinary professional and educational organization devoted to transgender health). Orchiectomy is performed as an outpatient surgery under local anesthesia with sedation, or under general anesthesia.

Surgeons remove the testicles and spermatic cords by way of a midline incision in the scrotum. (Groin incisions on either side are not needed and create unnecessary scars. If your surgeon is nonnegotiable about this point, get another opinion.) Care is taken to minimize tissue loss, as the scrotal tissue is used in vaginoplasty. (The scrotum looks smaller after the testicles are removed because it is no longer distended by them.)

After orchiectomy, an individual no longer takes a testosterone blocker such as spironolactone or cyproterone acetate. This simplifies a trans woman's medical regimen and in the case of spironolactone, eliminates the diuretic effect.

Vaginoplasty

Vaginoplasty (basically, "building a vagina") goes by several names and will likely have more names in years ahead. **The current hot term is *gender-affirming vaginoplasty* (GAV).** But it is also commonly called gender-affirming surgery (GAS), gender-reassignment surgery (GRS), or sexual reassignment surgery (SRS). The term "sex change" is outdated.

Before getting into the details, it is important to mention just how far genital surgery has come. Years ago, surgical results were not nearly as elegant as they are today. In years past, trans women seeking genital surgery often had no choice but to sacrifice their sexual responsiveness.

In the 1980s when I transitioned, there was no easy way to find out if you had a good surgeon or not. There were no before-and-after pictures or reviews by former patients to fall back on. The surgeon my psychiatrist referred me to was my only choice. When the surgery was done, I was ecstatic!

When the swelling went down, I started to see the work he did in more detail and noticed that there was no clitoris, or none in the right place, and no real labia minora. When I went in for my next post-op checkup, I complained that my new vagina wasn't very anatomically correct, to which he replied, "Turn off the lights, nobody will notice."

I had no recourse or legal rights back then, so I had to bite my tongue.

— *Trans woman who transitioned in the 1980s*

While they might have had an acceptable genital appearance, many sacrificed the ability to orgasm. But because of advances in surgical techniques, trans women are now able to look and respond like the women they *are*. A good sex life should never be a "frill," so this is a significant development.

Let me explain how the newer surgeries have made sexual response possible.

Let's go back to embryology and how we developed before we were born. As embryos, our genitals grow from the same basic structures whether we are genetically male or female. The sensitive head of the penis (glans penis) is the embryologic equivalent of the natal female clitoris, although the clitoral head and shaft are much smaller. The natal scrotum is the embryologic equivalent of the labia majora in the natal female. And the perineal raphe (ridge) is analogous to the natal female labia minora. Note that these structures may be open or fused and yet still be analogous. Dr. Frank Netter's illustration in Figure 2.5 on page 47 color-codes these various structures, making it easier to understand which ones are analogous to others. So when the glans penis is transformed into a clitoris, the same neurologic pathways persist and sexual responsiveness is preserved.

While not shown in the Netter illustration, the testicles are analogous to the ovaries located deep in the female pelvis. Naturally, both genders have urethras to pass urine from the bladder to the outside of the body, and rectums through which the bowel movements travel to the outside world.

If you are not medically trained and do not speak medicine as a second language, stop for a moment before you go on. The following information about genital surgeries gets quite complicated. Don't get discouraged as you read. If you find this difficult, remember that it is complex information, but it is manageable.

It's *my* problem as the author if I cannot make it understandable! *Read slowly* and look up words you don't know.

— Linda Gromko, MD

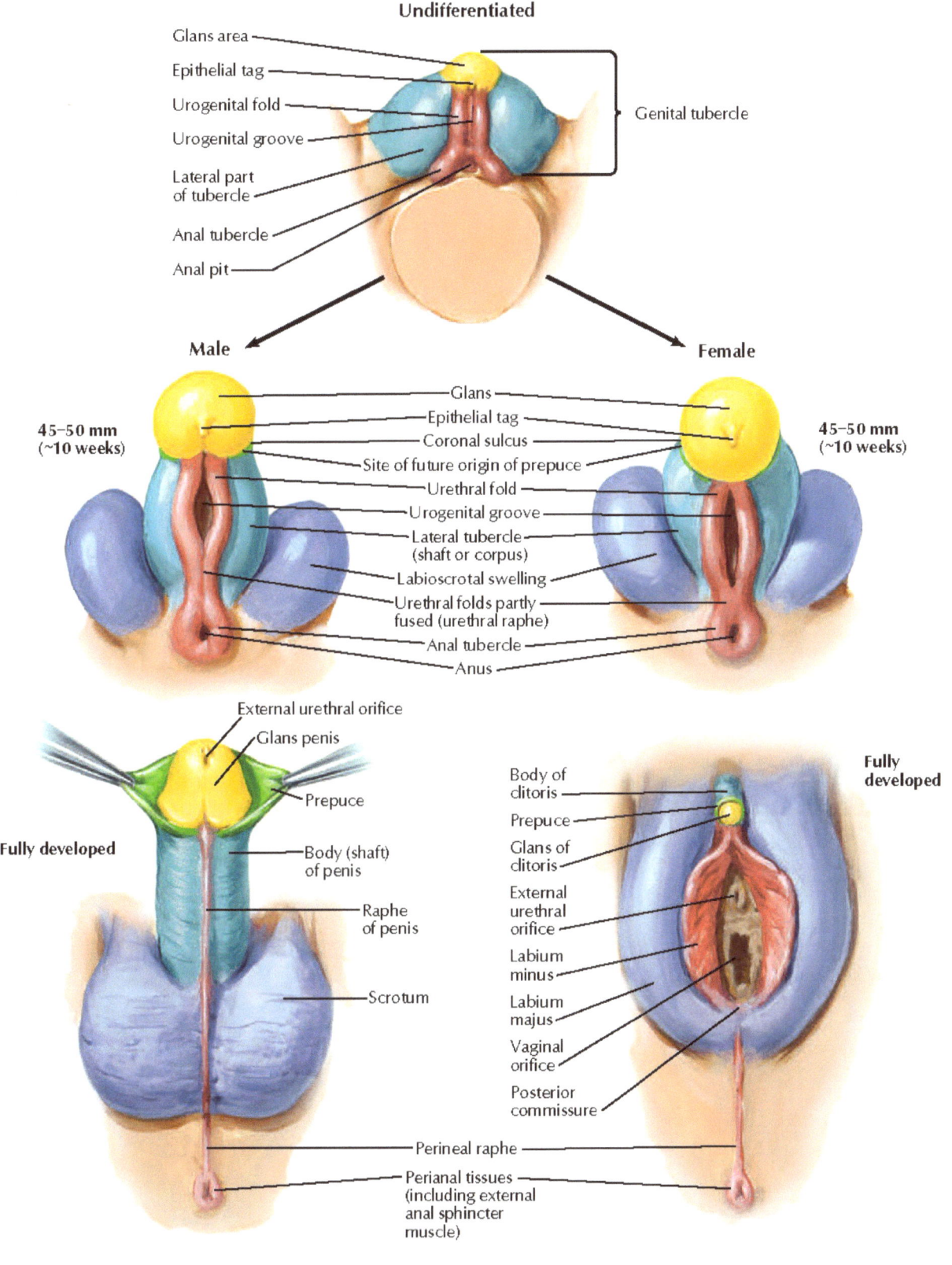

Figure 2.5. Embryologic equivalents in male and female external genitals.

Learning about the Feminizing Genital Surgeries

- Read the information out loud to another person or an animal. (I remember a medical school classmate who would tell her tiny daughter "stories" about the anatomy of the heart. Kids want to hear your voice and don't care as much about content.)

- Stop after every paragraph and be sure you're still on track before going ahead. Otherwise, you may get lost, anxious, and overwhelmed.

- Don't give up!

- If you're more of a visual learner, look at a picture, a medical illustration, a diagram, or a video. Visit YouTube (youtube.com) and search on the terms "sexual reassignment surgery," "vaginoplasty," or "MTF sex change."

Animation Videos of Vaginoplasty

Sexual reassignment (vaginoplasty) animation (youtube.com/watch?v=SH-j3r_Rwsw or youtube.com/watch?v=zGkiC3Y8kk0). While other sites show the actual surgery being performed, start here. It's simply illustrated, but it's still complicated. Know also that vaginoplasty techniques may vary, so start with these basics; they'll hold you in good stead.

Animation illustration by Rebecca Betts (youtube.com/watch?v=6J9-QORp8To). Most importantly, if you are reading this to prepare for your own surgery, be certain that you know exactly what you are having done. Speak to your surgeon, their ARNP or PA, the clinic coordinator, or someone else ("To whom may I talk with to get my questions answered before surgery?") Do not sign up for a surgery that you do not understand!

One-Stage Penile Inversion Vaginoplasty

Penile inversion vaginoplasty for gender affirmation was pioneered by surgeon Georges Burou in the 1950s and used more generally after his address to Stanford University in 1973. Early references to a "sensate vaginal pedicled spot" demonstrate earlier attention to sexual responsiveness.[19]

There are many variations in technique from surgeon to surgeon and from region to region. Obviously, a one-step vaginoplasty is designed to be completed at one time. In a two-step vaginoplasty, the hood of the clitoris and labia minora are completed during a second stage, usually several months later. (Some women do not go on to have Stage 2, as they are satisfied with their results of Stage 1.)

You may want to watch a YouTube animation as we go through the basics of the one-step procedure (youtube.com/watch?v=SH-j3r_Rwsw or youtube.com/watch?v=zGkiC3Y8kk0).

Or follow the medical illustrations of Hillary Wilson as you walk through the narrative below and on the next few pages. Remember that the procedure varies somewhat from surgeon to surgeon, but Wilson's color-coded illustrations will help you understand the basics.

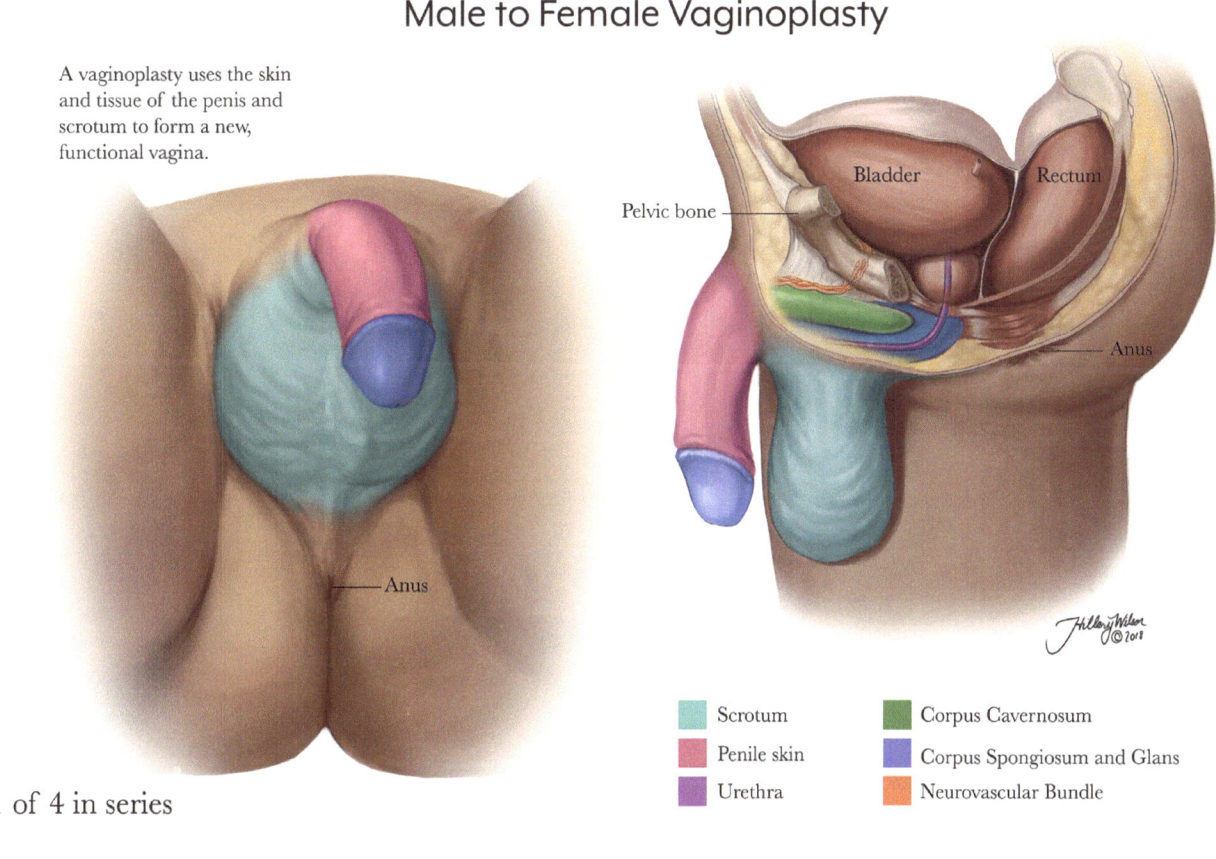

Figure 2.6. Vaginoplasty 1 of 4: The starting point.

---

19 Robert C. J. Kanhai, "Sensate Vagina Pedicled-Spot for Male-to-Female Transsexuals: The Experience in the First 50 Patients," *Aesthetic Plastic Surgery* 40, no. 2 (February 18, 2016): 284–7, https://doi.org/10.1007/s00266-016-0620-2.

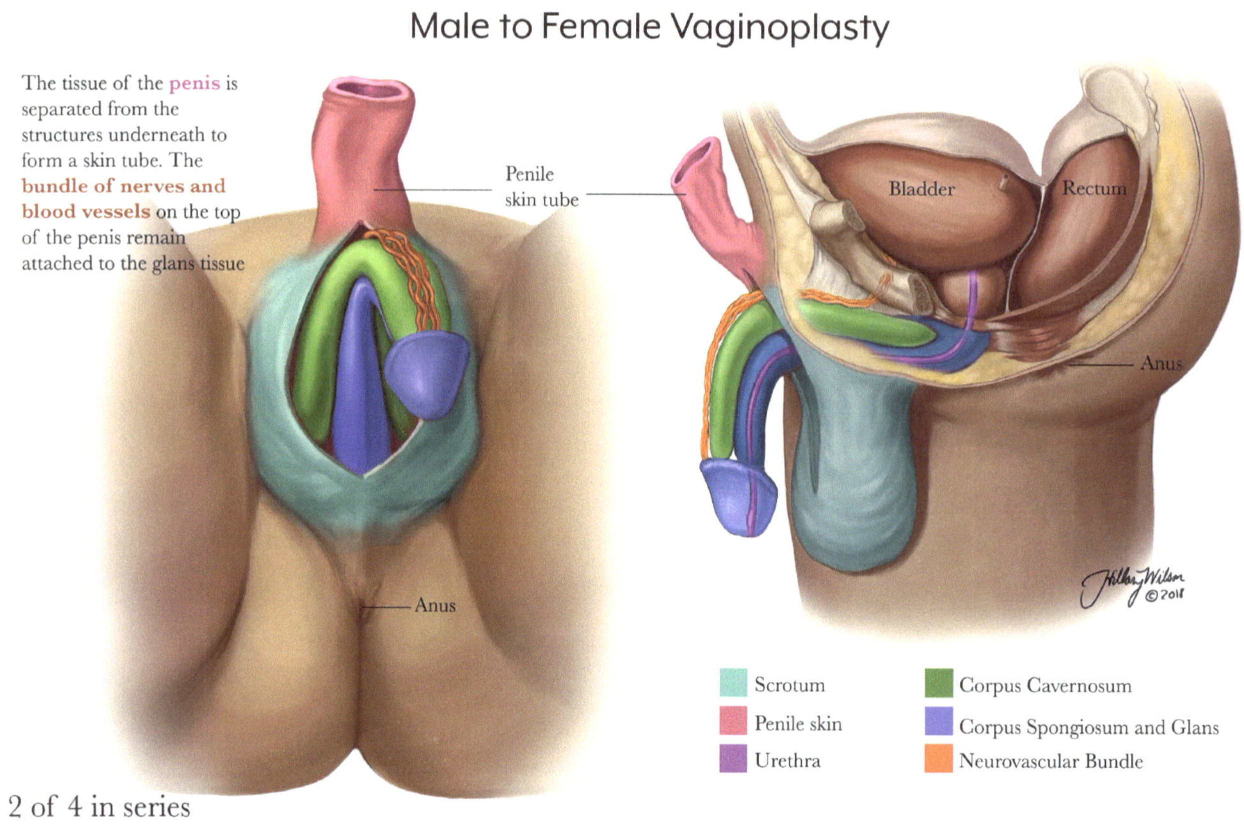

Male to Female Vaginoplasty

The tissue of the **penis** is separated from the structures underneath to form a skin tube. The **bundle of nerves and blood vessels** on the top of the penis remain attached to the glans tissue

Penile skin tube

Bladder

Rectum

Anus

Anus

- Scrotum
- Penile skin
- Urethra
- Corpus Cavernosum
- Corpus Spongiosum and Glans
- Neurovascular Bundle

2 of 4 in series

Figure 2.7. Vaginoplasty 2 of 4: The testicles are removed, and the penis is disassembled.

- The testicles are removed through an incision in the scrotum. ("Removed" means forever, which is why we emphasize sperm banking for fertility preservation before you even begin hormones or testosterone blockers.) The scrotal skin may be used to add more vaginal depth if needed, or to create the labia.

- The penis is dissected into its component parts. This is critical to retain urinary and sexual function. Here are the basic steps:

  - The skin of the penis is incised around the base of the glans (mushroom part). This skin is then pushed to the base of the penis. It will be inverted later and used to create the lining of neovagina (new vagina).

  - The neurovascular bundle—that is, the nerves, veins, and arteries that serve the glans penis—are dissected apart from the underlying structures. The neurovascular bundle remains attached to the glans penis at the dorsal surface.

  - The urethra is separated away from the cavernous bodies—the two pontoon-like structures that fill up with blood during an erection.

  - The corpora cavernosa or cavernous bodies are removed and discarded. To be precise, they are sent to the hospital's pathology department for examination and disposal (incineration).

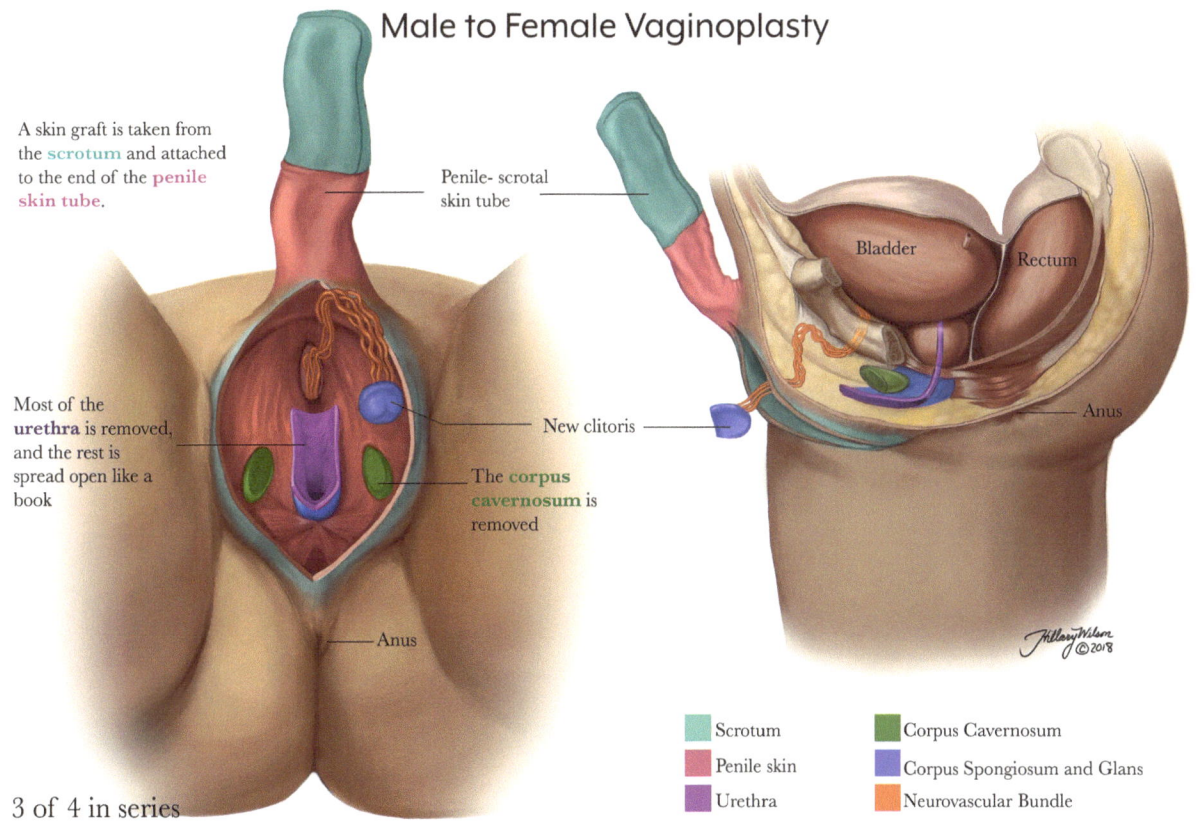

Figure 2.8. Vaginoplasty 3 of 4: The glans penis is reduced and reshaped to become the neoclitoris.

- The glans penis is reduced in size and rounded to become the neoclitoris, still keeping it as the sexual pleasure center. Because the nerves are still intact, stimulation of the neoclitoris will generally result in orgasm in people who had orgasms prior to surgery. Creating a clitoris of the "correct" size is important: if it is too small, the neoclitoris will be hard to find, and too large, it will look just like a small penis. Urine does not flow through the clitoris as it would in the penis. Rather, the urine will flow through the urethra, which will open below the clitoris.

- The urethra is shortened. Urethral tissue no longer needed for a shorter female urethra is splayed out to line the vaginal vestibule.

- The internal vaginal space is created by blunt dissection. This means that the tissue planes are separated with the surgeon's gloved fingers rather than scalpels, scissors, or cutting cautery. Other surgeons dissect the canal sharply using cautery or scissors. The vaginal space is created between the bladder and the rectum. (Said another way, the bladder, urethra, and prostate gland will remain in *front* of the space of the neovagina, and the rectum sits behind it.)

- The skin of the penis is inverted and directed into this newly created vaginal space. The inverted penile skin lines this space and is held in place by vaginal packing or is anchored to the ischium (part of the pelvic structure) or deep sacrospinous ligaments. In most cases, the inverted penile skin does not provide enough tissue for a vagina with adequate depth, so the surgeon uses scrotal skin as a graft at the apex of the canal.

- The inversion of the penis into the new vaginal canal begins the process of closing the surgical site. It brings the apex of the exposed surgical site down to join with the base of the surgical site, revising it from an open oval to a curved incision line.

Think about this carefully: The surface skin on the *outside* of the original penis becomes the lining skin on the *inside* of the vagina. It is different tissue than cisgender vaginal tissue in that it is not a mucous membrane and does not provide lubrication during sexual arousal. Added lubrication in the form of a surgical or personal lubricant (such as Surgilube, Slippery Stuff, Sliquid) will be needed during dilation or sexual penetration to prevent microtears that can make a person more susceptible to infection.

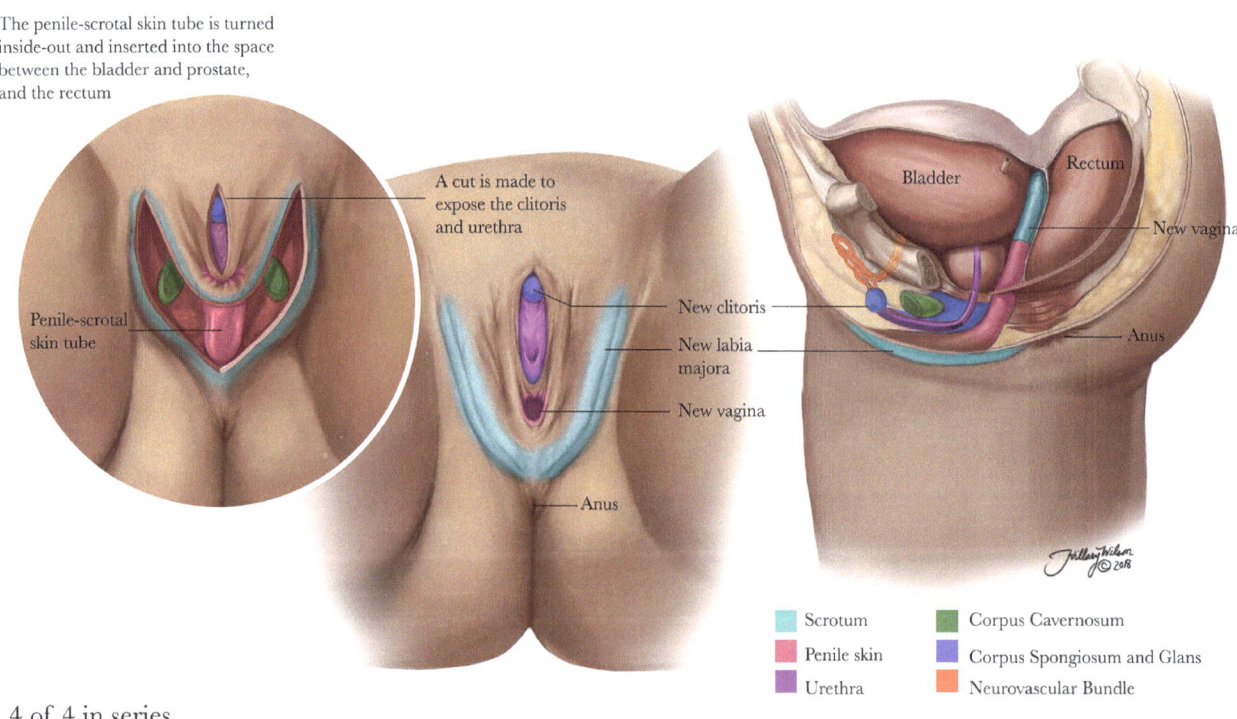

Figure 2.9. Vaginoplasty 4 of 4: Completion of the neovagina and creation of the labia.

- External openings in the skin below the pubic bone are created for the neoclitoris and for the urethra right below it. The urethra will appear slightly lower in position than in a natal female.

- Labia are created by using tissue from the inverted penis and the scrotum, depending on the technique being used. If the neoclitoris is not "hooded" at this time, it will be completed as part of Step 2 in a two-step procedure (Step 2 is also called a "labiaplasty").

After the vaginoplasty is completed, a urinary catheter is placed in the urethra and vaginal packing is inserted to minimize bleeding, to hold the neovagina in place, and to maintain vaginal patency (that is, to keep the vagina from closing in on itself). The catheter and vaginal packing are removed by the surgical staff about 5 to 7 days after surgery, marking the beginning of the routine of vaginal dilation to maintain vaginal depth and girth. (See pages 120–123 in Chapter 6).

What Happens to the Prostate?

The prostate gland is left in its original location, "wrapped" around the urethra at the base of the bladder. It is generally smaller after exposure to estradiol, so an enlarged prostate in a trans woman could be worrisome. The examiner palpates (feels) the prostate through the vagina; it is just on the other side of the anterior (front) vaginal wall. When examining a male, I palpate the prostate during a rectal exam. With my patient leaning forward over an exam table, I feel the prostate through the rectum, and just on the other side of the anterior (front) wall of the rectum.

Two-Stage Vaginoplasty
(Penile Inversion Vaginoplasty plus Labiaplasty Done Later)

Some surgeons perform vaginoplasty as a two-step procedure, with the second stage performed about 3 to 4 months after the initial vaginoplasty.

Not all clients go on to have the second stage performed, as they may be fully satisfied with the initial vaginoplasty results. However, the labiaplasty may increase a woman's comfort, particularly if the exposed neoclitoris protrudes to the extent where it is irritating.

Labiaplasty allows a surgeon to refine thinner labia minora and to create a more defined hood over the clitoris. A vertical incision is used in the procedure. Labiaplasty can be done as a day surgery. If there are other refinements or revisions to be done, these can be performed at the time of the labiaplasty.

> If you look up the word "labiaplasty," you are likely to find information about a cosmetic procedure to improve the appearance or tightness of a vagina. It is sometimes advanced as a treatment for rejuvenating the aging natal vagina. This is a different category of labiaplasty altogether, and the two are not performed for the same reasons.
>
> — Linda Gromko, MD

The Limited-Depth or Zero-Depth Vagina

Limited-depth vaginoplasties are also known as zero-depth vaginoplasties or vulvoplasties. (The term "vulva" refers to the external genitalia, including the labia majora and minora. You will notice that I often use the term "vagina" to refer to these structures—and this is not really accurate. "Vagina" refers to the internal genital structure. I am aware of this, but I use "vagina" because it is better understood and therefore communicated more clearly.)

Particularly for women who do not plan to have vaginal penetration, a limited-depth procedure provides for the removal of penis, scrotum, and testicles; the creation of a neoclitoris and labia; and the relocation of the urethra. In essence, the limited-depth vagina looks like that of an assigned female except that there is no vaginal "vault." Sometimes, a small depression or dimple is created. A limited-depth vagina allows a woman to urinate like other females and to orgasm since she has a functional clitoris.

Hair removal may not be required prior to the limited-depth vaginoplasty, but confirm this with your surgeon. Vaginal dilation is not needed.

As the surgery itself is less lengthy, a limited-depth procedure may be an excellent option for a woman with medical factors that would make it more difficult for her to weather a more extensive vaginoplasty and recovery period.

Vaginoplasty with Limited Graft Tissue

In a penile inversion vaginoplasty, the neovagina is created from the inverted penis and often a graft derived from scrotal tissue.

Particularly with the use of puberty blockers in transgender adolescents, we are likely to see more young people coming to vaginoplasty with less genital tissue. If histrelin or a Lupron-Depot blockade is initiated in early puberty and the adolescent goes on to use cross-sex hormones, the penis and scrotum do not grow to full adult size.

Circumcision (the removal of infant foreskin that is done on most babies assigned male at birth in the United States) can also limit the amount of available skin.

Full- or partial-thickness grafts may be derived from the lateral flank or abdominal areas at the waist. In this technique, scars are concealed within the skin lines at the waist and covered by underpants or a swimsuit. It may also be possible to do a peritoneal pull-through vaginoplasty, where the peritoneal membrane from the abdomen is used to line the upper vaginal vault, or a colovaginoplasty, where colonic tissue forms the neovagina.

The Peritoneal Pull-Through Vaginoplasty

More recently, there has been the development of the peritoneal pull-through vaginoplasty technique. Dr. Davydov popularized this technique in the mid-twentieth century as a solution for cisgender women with vaginal agenesis (a birth defect involving the absence of or an incomplete vagina), and it is now also being used in gender-affirmation surgery.

After the same initial steps of the penile inversion technique, an abdominal procedure, which can be done laparoscopically or as a robot-assisted laparoscopic procedure, is performed to obtain peritoneal grafts that then line the neovagina and attach it to the epithelium at the perineum or lower vagina. All external genitalia and the vaginal opening are fashioned from penile and scrotal skin. The peritoneal graft can be used for a primary vaginoplasty, a secondary salvage vaginoplasty, or as an adjunct to penile inversion to add additional depth to the neovagina.

The risks include all those associated with the penile inversion technique—that is, possible stenosis (narrowing of the opening) and graft rejection—as well as those with abdominal laparoscopic surgery. In cisgender women with vaginal agenesis, the benefits include some natural lubrication, less need for dilation, less need for douching, and adequate depth. There are currently no data on long-term outcomes for the peritoneal grafting procedure in transgender individuals.

— Heidi Wittenberg, MD

In the peritoneal pull-through procedure or series of procedures, an individual first undergoes an orchiectomy (removal of the testicles). A vaginal vault is developed in the perineum and lined with a portion of the *peritoneal* membrane that encloses the abdominal organs. This tissue is brought down from the abdomen by way of robotic-assisted laparoscopy. Here, the peritoneal membrane becomes the lining of the neovagina.

Alternatively, in the full-thickness skin graft technique, a graft is typically taken from the abdomen and used as the lining for the vaginal canal. The skin graft is harvested using an abdominoplasty incision (a horizontal incision like you would see with a tummy tuck). The advantage of this approach, of course, is that you can get a tummy tuck at the same time. The disadvantage, when compared to the peritoneal-pull through, is the presence of a potentially long horizontal scar on the abdomen. Scrotal tissue is used to form the vaginal labia.

Perineum versus Peritoneum: Big Difference!

According to the Merriam-Webster dictionary, the perineum is "the area between the anus and the posterior part of the external genitalia." It is also defined as "an area between the thighs that marks the approximate lower boundary of the pelvis and is occupied by the urinary and genital ducts and rectum." (We sit on our perineums.)

The peritoneum, on the other hand, is an internal abdominal membrane that consists of two layers: the parietal peritoneum that lines the abdominal and pelvic cavities, and the visceral peritoneum that encloses the stomach, most of the small and large intestines, and the liver, gallbladder, and spleen.

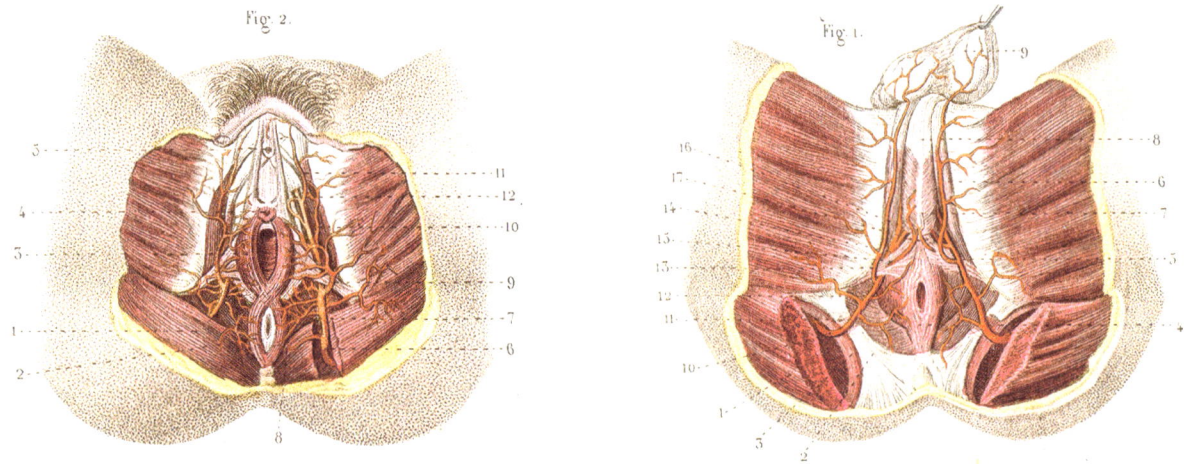

Figure 2.10. The perineum in an AFAB (left) and an AMAB (right).

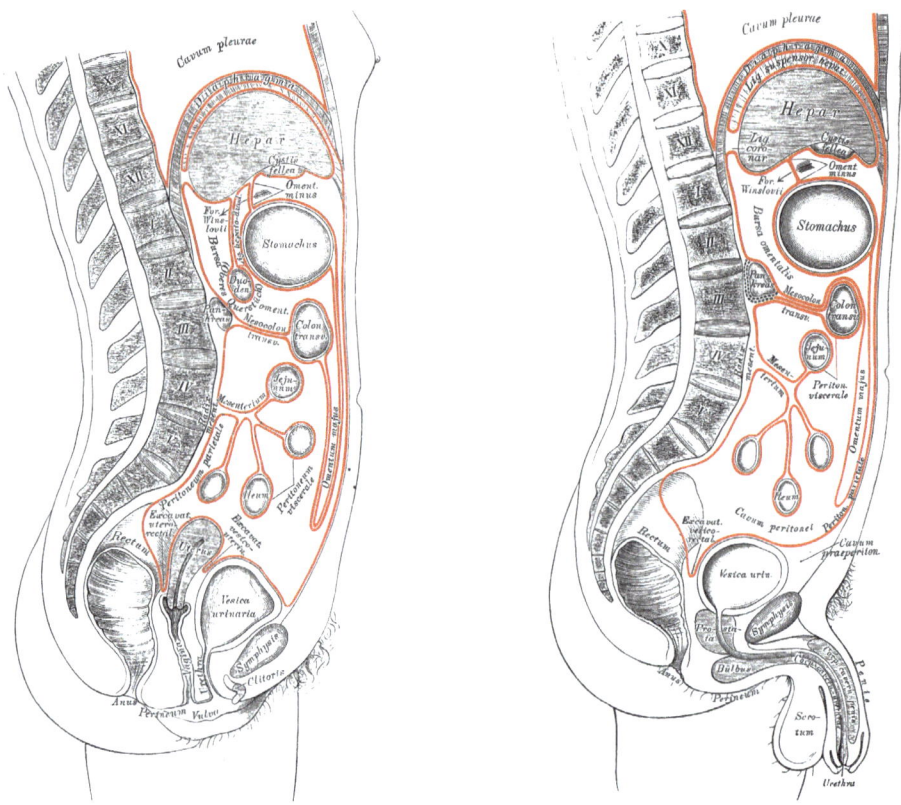

*Figure 2.11. The peritoneum in an AFAB (left) and an AMAB (right).
Trace the peritoneal membrane as it encloses the various abdominal organs (red lines).
The peritoneum consists of two layers, with a "potential space" in between.*

In AFAB individuals, the fallopian tubes and ovaries are included within the visceral peritoneum. The top of the uterus indents the peritoneum but is not enclosed by it. The kidneys, the upper part of the ureters, adrenal glands, the aorta, and the inferior vena cava are retroperitoneal. This means that these organs sit behind the peritoneal membrane and are not enclosed by it.

The parietal and visceral peritoneum lie immediately on top of each other, but can glide over each other since they're lubricated by secretions containing water, protein, and electrolytes. The area between the peritoneal layers is referred to as a "potential space." It is normally not a space at all, but it can be filled by pus, blood, or other fluid in states of infection, trauma, or malignancy.

For information on the penis/phallus-preserving vaginoplasty, refer to the newer nonbinary options below and on the next several pages.

Vaginoplasty Using the Sigmoid Colon (Rectosigmoid Vaginoplasty)

The rectosigmoid vaginoplasty[20] is rarely used in the United States, except in "salvage" or reconstructive surgeries in the event of vaginoplasty complications. First performed in 1904, the use of sigmoid and rectal tissue to create the neovagina has theoretical appeal for several reasons:

- The sigmoid colon self-lubricates with mucus.

- The length of the vagina created is not limited by the length of the penis (although this is circumvented by using scrotal or other tissue).

- Hair removal is not required preoperatively.

- Rectosigmoid surgery can now be done laparoscopically or robotically; in the past, an abdominal incision was required.

However, rectosigmoid surgeries have disadvantages as well:

- The lubrication produced by the sigmoid colon is *very* abundant.

- Colonic lubrication is continuous.

- Colonic secretions may have an associated odor.

- The neovagina still requires dilation.

- Dehiscence (the spontaneous opening of sutures) of the colonic repair can occur and may have life-threatening complications such as sepsis (bloodstream infection) or necrotizing fasciitis.

- The vaginal opening may look like colon tissue, even resembling a stoma in a colostomy rather than labia. This is not correctable by plastic surgery.

- Prolapse (out-pouching of the neovagina) can occur, but it is correctable.

- Screening an individual for colon cancer would require examining the neovagina as well as the colon; otherwise a colon cancer could go undetected.

Rectosigmoid vaginoplasty is widely used throughout the world, although penile inversion vaginoplasty has surpassed it in popularity.

---

20 "Bowel vaginoplasty was first described by Sneguireff in 1892 using the rectum in the treatment of vaginal agenesis. Later, in 1904, Baldwin reported the use of ileal segment in the treatment of congenital vaginal absence, but also suggested that the sigmoid colon might be used for the same purpose... In male to female transsexuals, first mention of intestinal vaginoplasty dates from 1974, when Markland and Hastings used cecum and sigmoid transplants." Marta Bizic et al., "An Overview of Neovaginal Reconstruction Options in Male to Female Transsexuals," *The Scientific World Journal* 2014, Article ID 638919 (May 26, 2014): 8 pages, https://doi.org/10.1155/2014/638919.

Vaginoplasty Using the Right (Ascending) Colon: aka Right Colo-Vaginoplasty

Note: Information about this surgery is provided by Geoffrey Stiller, MD.

See Figure 2.12 below. As you look at the drawing, remind yourself that the "right colon" refers to the *patient's* right. Remember that the ascending colon begins with the cecum, which is where the appendix originates. The stool is liquid when it moves from the small intestine into the cecum and ascending colon. It then travels upward to the hepatic (liver) flexure, where the colon turns at a near-right angle and travels horizontally to the splenic (spleen) flexure on the left side of the body. The colon takes another near-right angle turn as it becomes the descending colon and ultimately, the sigmoid and rectum.

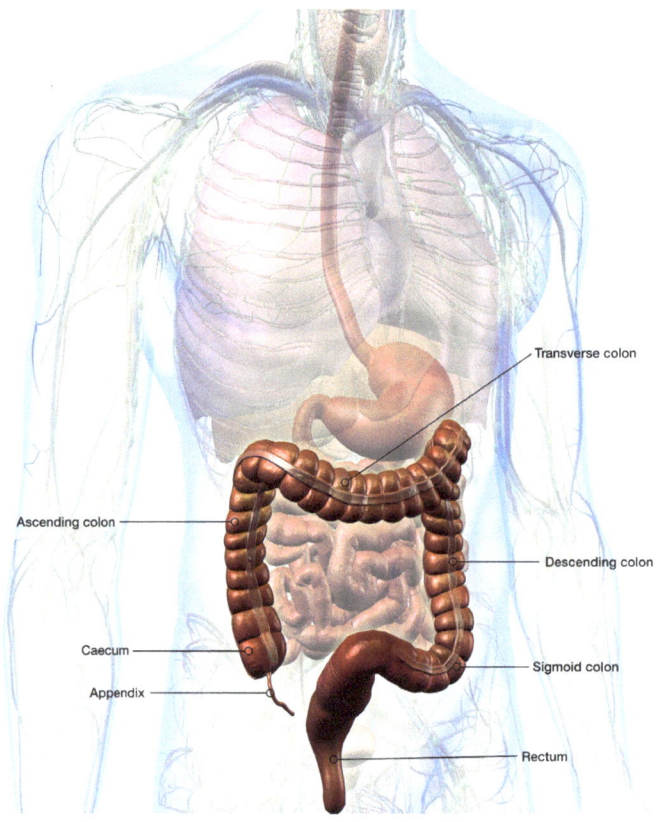

Figure 2.12. Anatomy of the colon.

The main function of the colon is to absorb fluid from the liquid stool, transferring it as a solid stool to the sigmoid colon and rectum—from which it is eliminated.

Another—and newer technique for vaginoplasty—uses the right or ascending colon rather than the sigmoid colon to create the vaginal vault. The right-colon vaginoplasty is offered as a primary procedure as well as a salvage operation for the revision of complications.

Right-colon vaginoplasty may be done in two separate surgeries. The first surgery is the creation of a zero-depth vagina using penile and scrotal tissue to create the labia. After a recovery period, the patient returns for the creation of the vaginal vault. Here, the right colon is moved to join the perineum at what will become the opening to the neovagina.

Because the full right colon is mobilized, vaginal depth can be generous (such as 9 inches), regardless of the patient's penile and scrotal size. The mobilization of the right colon can be done laparoscopically.

Potential Advantages of the Right-Colon Vaginoplasty

- The size of the right colon allows for a generous neovaginal depth, regardless of penile and scrotal size. This may be helpful in patients who are less well endowed, including those individuals who had puberty blockers and thus developed a smaller volume of genital tissue.

- The appendix can be removed at the time of this surgery, eliminating it as a potential site of inflammation (appendicitis) in later life.

- The blood supply of the right colon is generous, since several branches of the mesenteric vessels feed it. The sigmoid colon has a more complex arterial network with shorter branches.

- The colonic tissue is moved to the vaginal site, carrying its blood supply with it.

- No electrolysis is needed preoperatively, as the penis and possibly part of the scrotum are not inverted to create the internal tissues of the neovagina. This means no hair in the neovagina! We recognize that genital hair removal is expensive and time-consuming and can be painful.

- Using the penis and scrotum for the vaginal labia may result in a superior cosmetic result; simply, there is more tissue to use.

- The right colon lubricates, providing lubrication for the neovagina.

- If a patient is satisfied with Step 1—the creation of the zero-depth vagina—she can stop there.

Potential Disadvantages

- There are usually two surgeries, with exposures to two rounds of anesthesia. Two hospitalizations can mean more cost and more exposure to nosocomial infections (infections that a person contracts in the hospital, perhaps from sturdier, more drug-resistant bacteria).

- There may be an odor for roughly 6 months.

- Screening for colon cancer may become more complex. In a screening colonoscopy, a scope is introduced via the rectum so the examiner can see all the way along the colon to its beginning— that is, the cecum of the right colon. If a portion of the right colon becomes the neovagina, the vagina must also be scoped to perform a full exam of the colon.

> I would prefer that a colonoscope was used for screening; however, if a vaginal speculum can expose the entire vagina, that may be fine. If my patients have a hard time finding a gastroenterologist who is comfortable doing a vaginal scope at the time of their colonoscopy, then I would be more than happy to do their colonoscopy.
>
> — *Geoffrey Stiller, MD*

Dr. Alvaro H. Rodriguez Introduces Vaginoplasty Grafts from Tilapia at the WPATH 26th Scientific Symposium Surgeon's Program

Tilapia is the common name for a species of freshwater fish that is farmed all over the world. Plentiful and inexpensive, Nile tilapia were first used to graft burn injuries in human and animal skin in Brazil in 2015.

At the WPATH 26th Scientific Symposium Surgeon's Program on November 7, 2020, Dr. Alvaro H. Rodriguez presented a new use for tilapia—as a graft in vaginoplasty.[21] Rodriguez, a Colombian reconstructive surgeon specializing in gender-affirmation surgery and creator of the technique, stated,

> "After several years of research, we found that tilapia skin shares the same type of collagen as human skin, and it has almost the same strength. Because it is a fish, tilapia has DNA that is different than in humans. We think that is why tilapia skin is not rejected by human tissue."

Rodriguez went on to explain that after grafting the tilapia to line the neovagina, the tilapia skin is absorbed completely, leaving only the collagen.

> "This works as a matrix for the growth of new epithelium that looks like the vaginal mucosa both macroscopically and histologically."

Rodriguez showed pictures of tilapia skin with a prominent scale pattern. He explained that the fish skin is prepared by sterilization to be sure it is free of bacteria, and that the scales leave a tattoo pattern on the skin even though the scales themselves do not remain.

Dr. Rodriguez and colleagues are preparing their results for publication and are examining other uses of tilapia grafts that may serve the transgender community. Read more about Dr. Rodriguez's research and contact him at cecmcolombia.com.

In addition to Dr. Rodriguez, the tilapia research was conducted by Universidade Federal do Ceará professor Edmar Maciel Lima Júnior MD, coordinator of the research and head of the studies on the use of tilapia skin for burn treatment at the Instituto José Frota in Fortaleza, Ceará, Brazil, as well as Universidade Federal do Ceará professor Leonardo Bezerra PhD, coordinator of research in gynecology. Dr. Bezerra is also a pioneer of the treatment of vaginal agenesis (Mayer-Rokitansky-Küster-Hauser syndrome) with tilapia skin xenograft.

---

21 Alvaro H. Rodriguez, "Male-to-Female Gender Affirming Surgery Using Nile Tilapia Fish Skin as a Biocompatible Graft," (presentation, WPATH 26th Scientific Symposium Surgeon's Program, November 7, 2020).

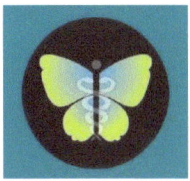

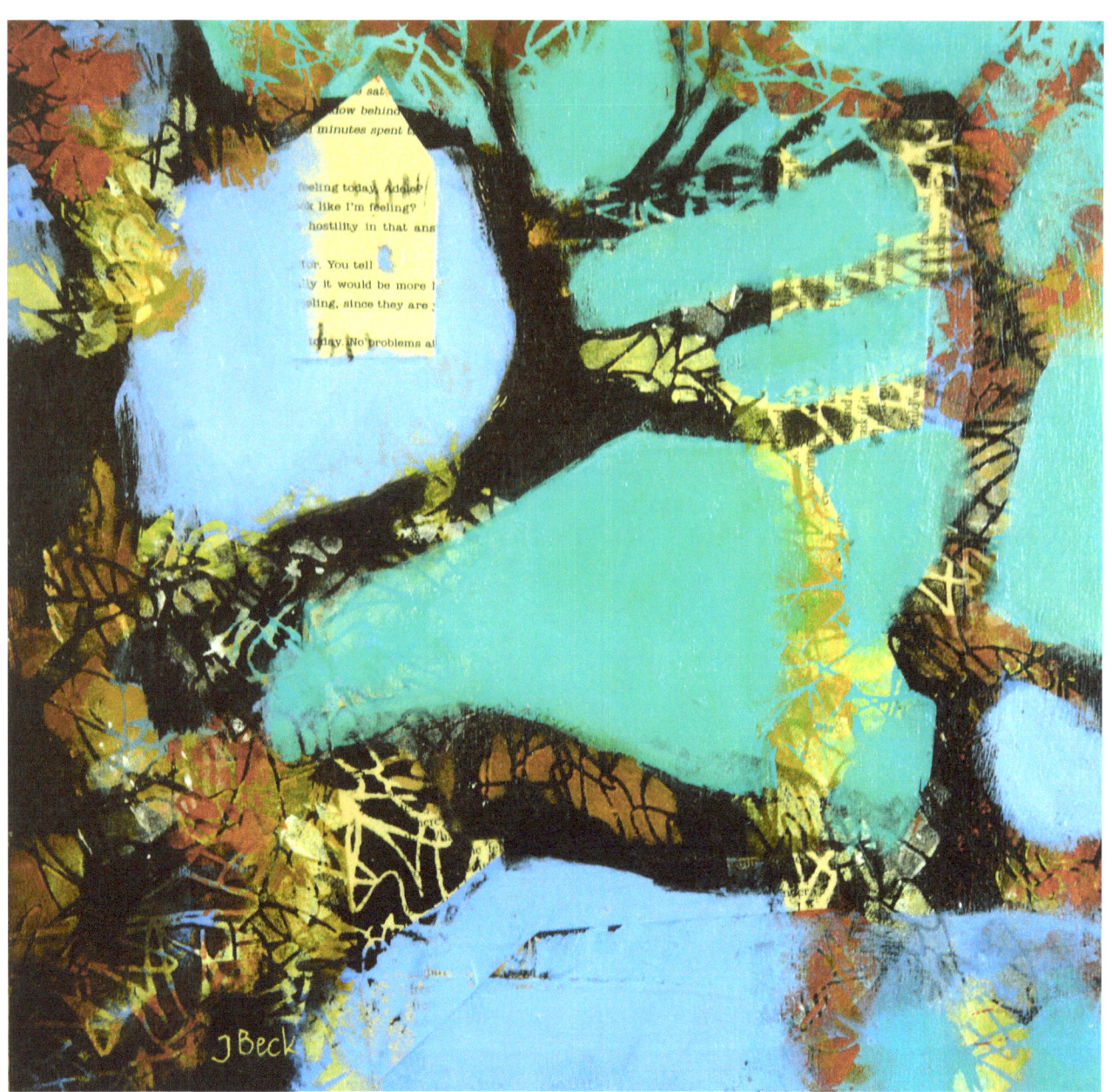

Birdhouse

CHAPTER 3
Masculinizing Surgeries

> ### Disclaimer
>
> The information provided here is intended to give you an overview on gender-affirming surgeries. It is not intended as medical advice for you personally.
>
> ***For medical advice pertaining to you specifically, seek your answers from your surgeon and their surgical team.*** They are the obvious professionals who will have the answers pertaining to your body and your circumstances. Information provided by them must be given more weight than my input. You will also note that I am not including photos of surgical outcomes. They are widely available on the websites of the surgeons.

Facial Masculinization Surgery

A first case of *full* facial masculinization surgery (FMS) was performed by Dr. Jordan Deschamps-Braly in 2015. Many of the techniques used resemble FFS in reverse, but Deschamps-Braly also introduced the technique of the Adam's apple implant using a cartilage graft from the patient's rib.

The rib cartilage is harvested through an inframammary incision, below the breast. The cartilage is then shaped to resemble a Y and implanted over and slightly below the patient's existing thyroid cartilage. Two notable points: (1) The rib cartilage is harvested via an *inframammary* incision that many trans men already have from top surgery, and (2) the cartilage graft is autologous, meaning that the patient will not reject their own grafted tissue.[22]

In more recent years, the practice of facial masculinization surgery has expanded, both in cis and trans males. As with FFS, facial masculinization surgeries represent an aggregate of separate procedures done together or in stages. Performed together, these surgeries may take 6 to 12 hours to perform.

You may want to review the part on facial feminization surgery earlier in this chapter to examine the basic differences between AFAB and AMAB faces. Generally, male faces have more prominent brow bones and larger, more angular jaws. Male-pattern hairlines appear squarer and more angular, particularly at the temples.

A typically "male" feature is the Adam's apple (thyroid cartilage), and it does not usually enlarge with the addition of testosterone in transition. Trans men do show facial changes while on testosterone. Some changes are likely due to a change in fat distribution, age, and changing hair patterns.

While others disagree, I believe bony changes are visibly evident also. I see it in our trans male patients, and you'll see some impressive chronologies on YouTube. I did not find scholarly documentation for facial bony changes in trans men on testosterone, but bone is living tissue and it does undergo remodeling.

---

22 Jordan C. Deschamps-Braly et al., "First Female-to-Male Facial Confirmation Surgery with Description of a New Procedure for Masculinization of the Thyroid Cartilage (Adam's Apple)," *Plastic & Reconstructive Surgery* 139, no. 4 (April 2017): 884e, https://doi.org/10.1097/prs.0000000000003185.

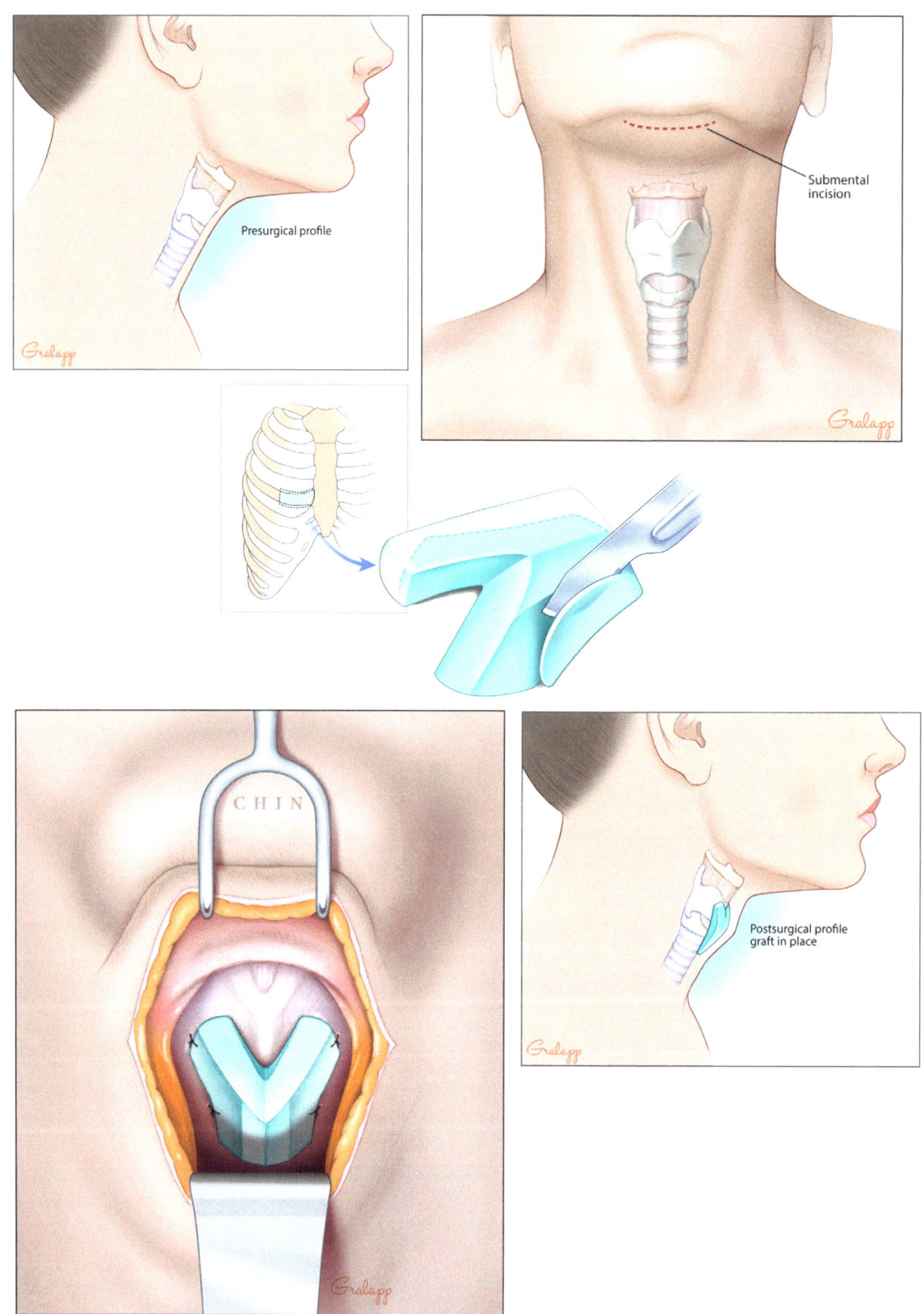

Figure 3.1. Tracheal augmentation.

As in FFS, your surgeon will want to know *your* desired outcomes. What would *you* like to see happen to enhance your facial masculinity? The surgeon will examine your head shape, hairline, face, and neck and offer their recommendations. It's important to remember that a single change in one part of the face will impact not only the appearance of adjacent structures, but the entire face. Because of the facial subtleties of gender, it is wise to seek out a surgeon with experience with transgender individuals.

FMS Is a Collection of Surgeries

In facial masculinization surgeries, you may see the following modifications:

- **Brow bone enhancement**
  The male brow bone is typically prominent (referred to as brow "bossing"). In FMS, the brow bone is augmented with implants or sculpted with a biologically completable chemical to create a ridge above the brow.

- **Forehead elongation**
  Male foreheads tend to appear higher, with more distance between the brows and from the brow to the hairline. In FMS, a higher forehead can be accomplished by lifting and moving the scalp backward, placing an implant between the brows, and revising the orbital sockets.

- **Hair transplants**
  Hair is harvested from the base of the skull, often one to three follicles at a time. The transplants fill in areas of androgynous alopecia (male pattern hair loss). But, do remember that balding is almost always read as male.

- **Rhinoplasty**
  This surgery, otherwise known as a nose job, creates a larger, more masculine-appearing nose. A male nose tends to be longer and not as upturned as a female nose. Rib cartilage can be used to enlarge the bridge of the nose or extend its length. Most importantly, the nose must balance the face.

- **Cheek implants**
  Implants accent the cheekbones. Implants imply that silicone or some other compatible material is inserted, while grafts are transfers of fat or bone from other parts of the body.

- **Chin and mandible contouring**
  The chin may be squared by lengthening it, and the angles of the jaw are made more prominent with a custom implant. The jawbones can be accessed from inside the mouth. Some surgeons make an exterior incision, such as under the chin, so it can be hidden.

- **Adam's apple enhancement**
  Although both males and females have an Adam's apple (thyroid cartilage), it is typically much more prominent in natal males. As stated earlier, Dr. Jordan Deschamps-Braly described his technique of harvesting and shaping rib cartilage and placing it over the existing thyroid cartilage to create a visible Adam's apple. The harvest of the rib cartilage is made at the inframammary crease, often through an existing scar from top surgery.[23]

---

23 Deschamps-Braly et al., 884e.

- **Facelift**

  As in females, excess skin is removed and the lower and middle parts of the face are tightened to provide a more youthful appearance. However, if done in the same way as female faces, it may actually feminize the face. The techniques vary with males and should be approached in the same way as in cis men. Again, it is important to choose a surgeon who is expert in transgender facial variations. Incision lines may be camouflaged immediately in front of the ears or behind them. This is commonly done in middle-aged and older individuals.

Gender-Affirming Chest Reconstruction (Top Surgery)

Nothing seems to impact the overall life experience of individuals seeking to masculinize like top surgery does. It is a commonly performed surgery that is frequently covered by insurance (sometimes even in adolescents), and it grants trans men freedom from wearing chest binders.

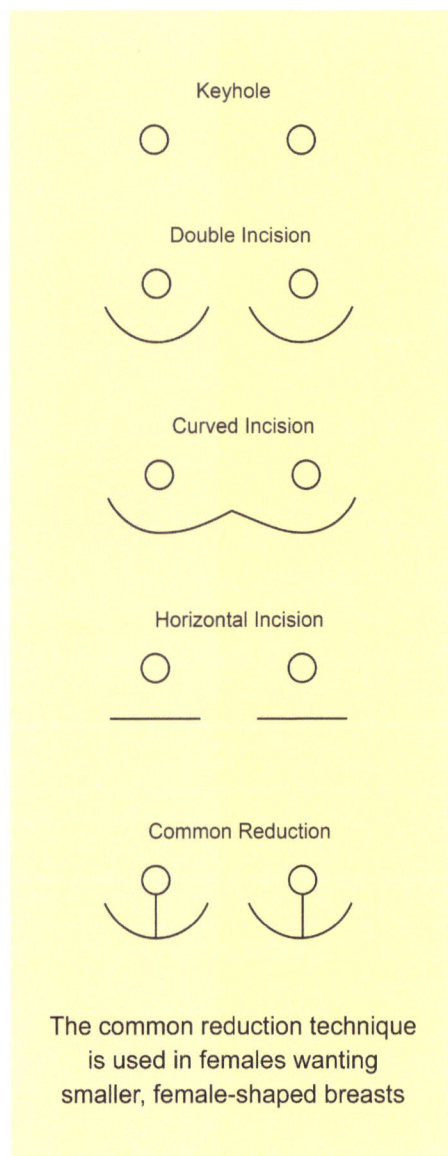

Figure 3.2. Top-surgery scars.

The goal of top surgery is to create a *male* chest contour, not to create *smaller female-appearing* breasts. Look at the diagram at left to see the differences between the scars after a reduction mammoplasty and typical gender-affirming top surgery.

Postsurgical Scars in Reduction Mammoplasty versus Top Surgery

There are two general types of top surgeries, and they both depend on the size of the breasts before surgery.

Most trans men will have a *double incision surgery*. The double incision refers to the two nearly horizontal or curvilinear scars that follow the borders of the pectoralis muscles. In the double incision technique, most of the breast tissue is removed, while some remains to create a masculine contour. Sometimes, instead of having two separate incisions, the double incisions are connected into a single curvilinear incision. The effect of each type of top surgery is to create the appearance of a "cut" (fit or "buff") pectoralis muscle.

In the double incision surgery, the areolas (or more properly, the nipples and areolas) are removed and reshaped. (Aerolas are the colored parts around the nipples.) Male areolas are considerably smaller than female areolas. The nipple and areolar complex are grafted back onto the chest at the end of the surgery, and a medicated gauze stent or bolster is sewn on to secure the areola. After about 5 to 7 days, the nipple stents are removed. The nipple grafts must be kept moist with petroleum jelly or Aquaphor for the next 2 weeks. By the time the stents are removed, the blood supply from the chest is serving the reattached nipple directly. This is a critical step and the reason surgeons are so insistent that a patient does not smoke.

> A surgeon told one of my clients:
> "If you don't stop smoking, your nipples may fall off like dried cornflakes."
>
> — Linda Gromko, MD

> What about nipples? At a 2021 WPATH Conference section dealing with gender nonbinary surgical enhancements, it was brought up that some clients are seeking top surgery without the reconstruction of nipples. People who are interested in this option should ask their surgeon; chest reconstruction without nipples is now considered an option by a number of surgeons.
>
> — Linda Gromko, MD

Areolar pigmentation may change in the process of top surgery. The areolas may appear mottled, with patches of hypopigmentation or even no pigmentation. Sometimes the nipple itself will not protrude as prominently as a patient might have hoped. Time and patience can remedy both of these conditions. Pigment often returns to the areola slowly over time. If all areas have not filled in by a year or two, tattooing may be used to fill in the hypopigmented (pink) parts. If the nipple projection is not enough, 3D tattooing can also be done using shading and highlights to create the appearance of a protruding nipple (see page 127).

Individuals who have less chest tissue may have keyhole surgery. For this surgery to be successful, the patient must have a relatively small amount of breast tissue and no excess skin. Additionally, the nipples and areolas must be small and they must naturally be positioned higher on the chest near the edge of the pectoralis muscle. If these requirements are not met, a person may have a more satisfactory result with a double incision procedure.

> What does a keyhole have to do with this? "Keyhole" is a confusing term as it implies a vertical incision so it looks like an old skeleton keyhole or a lollipop. Most surgeons have a different idea about what a keyhole approach actually is. It really should be called a periareolar or transareolar surgery.
>
> — Toby Meltzer, MD

With the keyhole technique, the surgeon enters the breast by making an incision under or around the areola. Most of the breast tissue is removed and the incision is sutured together. If the nipples are relatively large, they will be reshaped as in the double incision surgery.

As a reminder, top surgery does not eliminate the possibility of breast cancer, so chest exams done by a transmasculine person and their healthcare provider are important. Evaluation of any lump is critical, as is special attention to those men with cancer-provoking gene mutations such as BRCA1 and BRCA2.

Bidding the Girls—but Not My Personality—Goodbye

After top surgery, my level of self-confidence is amazing. I now walk with my head held high, but with a humble spirit. Because for me, stepping into manhood is NOT about going shirtless or so-called "masculine swag." It goes much deeper than that. It's becoming one with ALL of me. I'm finally embracing and celebrating ALL of who I AM: my Sacred Self; the wounded child; the strong-willed, fiercely independent but scarred woman; and the sensitive, soft-hearted man who isn't afraid of his feminine attributes. Becoming a man has allowed me to homogenize all of my Sacred Souls into that of a healthy, well-adjusted male.

Since taking this journey, I am being forced to confront all of my demons and embrace my quirks and flaws while opening my heart and mind to ongoing healing and growth.

Setting the Record Straight

Becoming a man wasn't about me finding "happiness" or peace of mind. I had to do the road work before entering the ring. Hence, after 4 years of weekly therapy, I was able to arrive at a place of psychological and emotional contentment BEFORE I was rolled into the surgical suite. This is because I've never believed top surgery and hormones to be a panacea or quick-fix—it was only to align my physical body with my inner truth.

So, What *Was* It All About?

My journey into manhood was not about being macho, chasing women, wearing three-piece tailored suits, finding happiness, escaping depression, hanging with the boys on a Saturday night, building large muscles, or gaining brawn. It's about acquiring emotional maturity, dignity under pressure, greater calmness in the midst of chaos, and gentleness and compassion toward myself and others. It's also about being accountable, having increased patience, having strength during those moments when I want to just let it all go, and pursuing continued spiritual development along with service to others.

For me, this is what becoming and being a man is all about. Have I arrived yet? Not yet, because I am a Designer's Original that is an ongoing work in progress.

— *Harlowe Rayne Thunderword-Cohen*

Hysterectomy and Bilateral Salpingo-Oophorectomy

Many—but certainly not all—trans men have their uterus, cervix, fallopian tubes, and ovaries removed.

Hysterectomy and bilateral salpingo-oophorectomy can be accomplished through the abdomen or the vagina. But today, these procedures are often done using minimally invasive surgical techniques such as laparoscopic and robot-assisted procedures. These enable the surgeon to make much smaller incisions. The organs are clearly seen, as a camera (the laparoscope) is placed through the belly button, and photographs are projected on large screens opposite the surgeon and assistant. In robotic surgeries, the surgeon actually manipulates the "hands" of the robot and the camera remotely via computer, while the assistant holds and retracts the laparoscopic instruments so the surgeon can see the surgical field.

> After the hysterectomy, I could feel that something was missing.
> But it was something that never should have been there in the first place.
>
> — *Trans man, age 55*

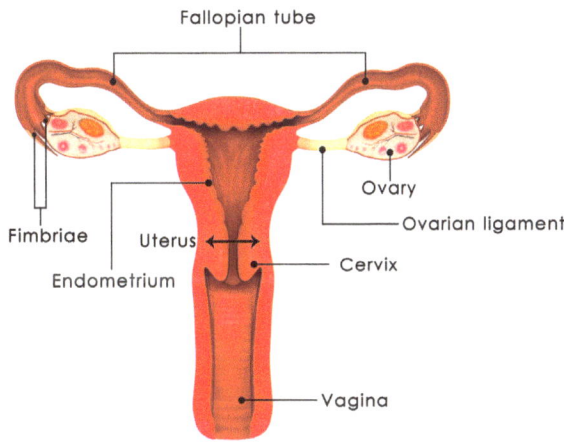

Figure 3.3. Internal female reproductive organs.

This surgery is done in preparation for phalloplasty, and removing these organs accomplishes the following:

- It allows for the definitive treatment of benign pathology, such as uterine fibroids, and essentially eliminates the possibility of cancer of the uterus, cervix, ovaries, or fallopian tubes. (Fallopian tube cancer is very rare but can occur in people who have the BRCA1 or BRCA2 gene mutation that also increases the risk of a person getting breast, ovarian, peritoneal, or pancreatic cancer.)[24] Typically, cancers of the ovary, fallopian tubes, or peritoneum have subtle symptoms that are recognized late in the disease process. Particularly for trans men who are reluctant to seek out gynecological care, removing these organs can be prudent.

---

24 Nancie Petrucelli, Mary B. Daly, and Tuya Pal, "BRCA1- and BRCA2-Associated Hereditary Breast and Ovarian Cancer," in *GeneReviews*, ed. Margaret P. Adam et al. (Seattle: University of Washington, 1993–2021, September 4, 1998), updated December 15, 2016, https://www.ncbi.nlm.nih.gov/books/NBK1247/.

- Eliminates the possibility of the vaginal bleeding that occurs when people run out of their testosterone, forget to take it, or are prescribed a dose that's too low. Bleeding can also occur due to a disease state, such as—and most importantly—with cancer. That's why bleeding that doesn't stop with hormone adjustments must be evaluated further.

A hysterectomy and bilateral salpingo-oophorectomy can be combined with procedures that reduce incontinence of urine or stool. This can be helpful for trans men who have had vaginal deliveries before transitioning.

Monsplasty

The mons pubis is a fatty area that lies over the pubic bone. It tends to be more prominent in assigned females, especially after having a baby, and there is no amount of physical exercise that can be done to get rid the mons specifically. It typically "reads" female. By liposuction or via an open horizontal incision, mons tissue is reduced to create a flat mons rather than a pooch. This surgery can be combined with other male reconstructive surgeries such as metoidioplasty or vaginectomy.[25]

Laparoscopy and Robot-Assisted Surgeries

Surgeries have changed a great deal over the past two decades. It used to be necessary for a surgeon to make an incision to see directly inside an exposed body cavity. Today, we are seeing the newer techniques of laparoscopy and robot-assisted surgery.

Q What is laparoscopy?

A In abdominal laparoscopy, three or four small incisions are made. One is to introduce a camera (the laparoscope) through the belly button; the other incisions create ports through which long-handled instruments are inserted. All the surgical "action" is projected from the umbilical camera onto two video screens—one facing the surgeon and the other facing the assistant. Rather than viewing the surgical field directly, the surgeon and assistant look at these screens while they manipulate instruments that are introduced through the ports.

Q What is robot-assisted surgery?

A Robot-assisted surgery is similar to laparoscopic surgeries in that small incisions are used to insert ports to access patient organs with long-handled instruments. But the surgeon sits at a console away from the patient and uses a computer to direct a robot's "hands," which in turn manipulate what's being operated on.

---

25   Osama Kamal Zaki Shaeer, "Shaeer's Technique: A Minimally Invasive Procedure for Monsplasty and Revealing the Concealed Penis," *PRS Global Open* 4, no. 8 (August 29, 2016): e1019, https://dx.doi.org/10.1097%2FGOX.0000000000001019. See also the video graphics at https://www.ncbi.nlm.nih.gov/pmc/articles/PMC5010356/figure/F9/.

Learning about the Masculinizing Genital Surgeries

> This is a repeat of information shared earlier: If you are not medically trained and do not speak medicine as a second language, stop for a moment before you go on. The following information about genital surgeries gets complicated. Don't get discouraged as you read. If you find this difficult, remember that it is complex information, but it is manageable. It's my problem as the author if I cannot make it understandable.
>
> — *Linda Gromko MD*

- Read slowly and look up words you don't know.

- Read the information out loud to another person or an animal. (I remember a medical school classmate who would tell her tiny daughter "stories" about the anatomy of the heart. Kids want to hear your voice and don't care as much about content.)

- Stop after every paragraph and be sure you are still on track before going ahead. Otherwise, you may get lost, anxious, and overwhelmed.

- Don't give up!

- If you're more of visual learner, look at a picture, a medical illustration, a diagram, or a video. Visit youtube.com and search on the terms "sexual reassignment surgery," "phalloplasty," "metoidioplasty," or "FTM sex change."

Most importantly, if you are reading this to prepare for your own surgery, be certain you know exactly what you are having done. Speak to your surgeon, the ARNP or PA, the clinic coordinator, or someone else in their office ("To whom may I talk with to get my questions answered before surgery?"). Do not sign up for a surgery you do not understand!

Masculinizing Genital Surgeries

Masculinizing genital surgery is also known as male sexual reassignment surgery, lower surgery, or bottom surgery. In this part, we will review the different types of masculinizing genital surgeries. Within each type, there are wide variations in style and technique. A phalloplasty, for example, may really incorporate three or four individual operations done in a series. These surgeries can be very complex, and surgical complications are not uncommon.

Male sexual reassignment surgeries have evolved tremendously over the past 20 years. Until recently, masculinizing genital surgeries were not covered by health insurance. Today, they are covered more commonly, particularly with larger group policies.

Each of the broader types of masculinizing surgeries has a different outcome—that is, it meets a different goal. It is critical that a person knows exactly what is important to them and to be clear about wanting genital surgery at all.

We have reviewed that embryonic genitals in assigned males and assigned females are virtually identical (refer to the Netter Embryologic Equivalents illustration on page 47 for a refresher). The clitoris and its shaft are the embryologic equivalent of the penis. Under the influence of testosterone, the clitoris enlarges and looks very much like a small penis. Many trans men find this clitoral enlargement (clitoromegaly) to be very satisfactory without *any* surgical intervention.

Certainly, many trans men don't want to risk the possibility of surgical complications. Many do not have financial access to surgery or regional access to a qualified surgeon. And I often hear from my clients, "I'm going to wait for another 10 years to see how these surgeries evolve."

Needless to say, it is important to do your homework. Talk to people who have had the various surgeries performed *on them*. Go to conferences, follow online groups, and explore reddit.com for candid information on trans male surgeries. Examine the photographs on the websites of various surgeons.

Deciding on the Best Type of Masculinizing Genital Surgery for You

Answer the Following Questions about Your Own Goals

- **Is it the *appearance* of my genitals that matters most to me?**
  (I'm told that many men really don't stare at one another's genitals in bathrooms or locker rooms, but surgery can make you feel more comfortable in these day-to-day situations.)

- **Is it important for me to have a *bulge* in my crotch?**

- **Is it important for me to have a scrotum?**

- **Is it important to have testicles that can be felt in the scrotum?**

- **Is it important that I am able to *stand* to pee?**

- **Is it important that I can pee *through* the end of my penis?**

- **Do I want to be able to use my penis to have sex with a partner?**
  Stated another way, is it important for me to be able to *penetrate* or enter my partner with my penis during sex? If so, am I seeking a particular size of penis?

Read through Table 3.1 below to help you sort out your own goals and match them to the various types of genital masculinizing surgeries available.

Deciding on a Type of Male Genital Surgery

Surgery Type	Looks like a Penis	Can Stand to Pee	Can Pee through the Penis	Can Use the Penis for Penetration	Bulge in the Crotch	Can Feel Testicles in the Scrotum
Metoidioplasty	Yes	Not through the phallus	No	No*	Unlikely	No
Metoidioplasty and urethral extension (lengthening)	Yes	Maybe**	Yes	No*	Unlikely	No
Metoidioplasty and scrotoplasty	Yes	Maybe with urethral extension**	With urethral extension	No*	Yes	No
Metoidioplasty and scrotoplasty and implants	Yes	Maybe with urethral extension**	With urethral extension	No*	Yes	Yes
Delayed pedicle flap phalloplasty only ("shaft only")	Yes***	No	No, unless modified with separate urethral lengthening	With an erectile pump	Yes	With scrotoplasty and implants
Phalloplasty with radial forearm or anterior thigh flap and urethral reconstruction	Yes	Yes	Yes	With a pump or malleable rod	Yes	With scrotoplasty and implants

Table 3.1. Deciding on a type of male genital surgery.

*   Metoidioplasty is generally not advertised for penetration, but many trans males state that they can penetrate partners. This is highly individual, so do not assume that penetration will be possible with metoidioplasty as you make your decision.

** Standing to pee is dependent on a person's overall size. If obese, a person may not be able to stand to pee after metoidioplasty with a urethral extension. A metoidioplasty phallus may not be long enough to clear a zipper, meaning that you may have to lower your pants to pee standing up.

*** Probably less "classic" appearance; can be modified.

Remember: You will not pee through a phallus without a urethral extension; nobody pees through a natal clitoris without urethral extension (urethral lengthening)!

Metoidioplasty (Also Known as "Meta")

The word *metoidioplasty* is derived from its Greek roots: *meta* (toward), *aidoia* (male genitals), and *plasty* (formation).

There are a number of variations on the metoidioplasty procedure, and which surgery a person selects depends on their overall goals.

In a basic metoidioplasty, the clitoris—which is already enlarged by the effects of testosterone—is released from its supporting ligaments. (Released, not removed!) The ligaments involved here are the suspensory ligament that connects the clitoris to the symphysis pubis (pubic bone) and the supporting ligaments of the labia minora. This type of metoidioplasty can also be called a "clitoral release." Tissue from the underside of the clitoris or the labia minora may be used to increase the "bulk" of the neophallus.

The effect of metoidioplasty is to make the clitoris appear longer, protrude farther, and look more penis-like. Metoidioplasty creates a phallus that measures about 4 to 6 centimeters. Given that 2½ centimeters equals 1 inch, you might have a phallus of about 2 inches in length. As stated above, sometimes girth *can* be augmented by using labial tissue.

Talk to your surgeon and be as specific as you can about what you want to see happen. Your surgeon should be able to give you an idea about how much length and girth you can expect. If you want to be able to pee through the penis, read on about metoidioplasty with urethral extension (urethral lengthening). Going back to embryology, nobody pees through the clitoris but assigned males pee *through* the urethral opening in the glans penis; so, the clitoris must be modified to make this possible.

Metoidioplasty with Urethral Extension (Also Called Urethral Lengthening)

Metoidioplasty with urethral extension is sometimes called a *metoidioplasty with a urethral hook-up*. The urethra (the tube through which you pee) is elongated and directed *through* the phallus. The skin used to elongate the urethra is often the buccal (pronounced "buckle") mucosa from inside the cheeks of the mouth, or skin from the inner lining of the vagina. This is a more complex procedure than metoidioplasty alone, and it has a greater risk of complications.

Other names may be used to describe various techniques. A ring metoidioplasty uses vaginal wall tissue and tissue from the labia minora to connect the urethra and the neophallus. The Centurion technique uses the round ligaments of the labia majora to add girth to the phallus. (See healthline.com/health/transgender/metoidioplasty.)

Any surgery that creates a new tube-like structure or elongates an existing one carries a risk for stricture, or narrowing of the newly created tube. The place where a new tube attaches to an existing one is called an "anastomosis" (connection). Anastomoses are particularly vulnerable to stricture or the formation of a fistula (an opening where it doesn't belong).

If a person has a stricture, he may be looking at several possible solutions, including dilation to widen the neourethra or a surgery to revise the urethral extension.

It is possible that a stricture can stop the urine flow entirely. The bladder continues to fill up with urine but the flow is obstructed. Should this happen, a man needs to be evaluated right away to dilate the stricture open and catheterize the urethra. If this cannot be accomplished, a suprapubic catheter can be inserted.

A man may require two catheters while the neourethra heals after surgery: one in the urethra and another placed in the suprapubic space that drains the bladder through the lower abdomen.

Q How does a man recognize that a stricture is developing?

A As the neourethra narrows, urine flow slows and it takes longer to pee. A man will also have to push harder to get the urine out.

Another complication of metoidioplasty with urethral lengthening is fistula formation. A fistula is a hole where there shouldn't be one—in this case, a new opening in the underside of the phallus. This causes dripping, or more than one urine stream appearing during urination. Fistulae may resolve spontaneously, or they may require a surgical repair. Today, because men who have had vaginectomies have significantly fewer fistulas and strictures, most surgeons do not perform urethral lengthening without vaginectomy.

A metoidioplasty with urethral extension enables a man to pee through the penis. It also allows a man to pee standing up, although this works best for trans men of normal body weight (not obese). As with trans women who have had a vaginoplasty, post-op trans men may have a urinary stream that may vary in direction for several months.

Metoidioplasty and Scrotoplasty with or without Testicular Implants

A scrotum can be created by fusing the labia majora in the midline. Adding well-vascularized fat grafts (fat has a rich blood supply) can add fullness to the neoscrotum. If a person elects, prosthetic testicles may be implanted into the neoscrotum. This gives more fullness and the appearance and feel of mobile testicles.

Sometimes, the scrotum is enlarged by placing tissue expanders in the neoscrotum to allow for larger testicular implants. Tissue expanders are fluid reservoirs that are placed temporarily within the scrotum. The owner injects gradually larger amounts of sterile water to gently stretch the tissue at designated time intervals. (Injection ports sit outside of the scrotum, so a man injects through the ports, not directly through his scrotal skin.)

Expectations for Metoidioplasty and Its Variations

These procedures provide for an excellent genital appearance. The phallus looks like a classic penis, although smaller. And in cases where the urethra is elongated and directed through the phallus, they allow for a trans man to pee standing up (although, as stated earlier, this works best for trans men who are not obese). Some men will have to lower their pants when urinating, as the phallus may not clear the zipper.

Metoidioplasties do not interfere with sexual sensation or orgasm. There is virtually no scarring, and recovery time is comparatively short. They can be combined with the more extensive procedures of hysterectomy (removal of the uterus), bilateral salpingo-oophorectomy (the removal of both ovaries and fallopian tubes), and vaginectomy (sealing of the vagina and closure of its perineal opening). These additions require more surgical time, a longer recovery, and more money.

If you are the kind of man who wants to keep his options open, know that you can have *all* the procedures described above, or even some of them, and still have a phalloplasty later on.

> One of my experienced trans male patients had a metoidioplasty and scrotoplasty several years ago. He was helping a younger trans man after his brand-new metoidioplasty and scrotoplasty.
>
> "Wow," said the younger one, "I can't believe I have a scrotum."
>
> "Yeah," said the veteran, "just wait 'til you get your balls!"
>
> — *Linda Gromko, MD*

Phalloplasty

Some Important Surgical Definitions

Knowing the difference between a graft and a flap is important in understanding these complex surgeries. Take your time to go through this information because it will make it much easier to comprehend what happens in the various phalloplasty techniques.

Skin Grafts and Flaps

Before we get into the details of phalloplasty, let's start by discussing the types of skin grafts and flaps that are used to build the neophallus (new penis). Grafts and flaps both serve the same two functions in phalloplasty: One function is to create the phallus itself; the other function is to physically cover the site where the penile graft or flap came from. This should become clearer in "Radial Forearm Flap Phalloplasty" starting on page 79 and the paragraphs that follow.

As you learn about grafts and flaps, refer to Figure 3.4, the anatomical illustration of the skin, on page 78 to further your understanding of the differences.

Definition of a Graft

In a graft, tissue is removed from one part of the body and reattached directly onto another site to cover a wound or a tissue defect from trauma. The donor site is the place where a graft is taken or removed. (The donor human and recipient human are the same person, so tissue rejection is not a problem.) **Grafts must rely on the blood supply at the site of attachment,** as opposed to flaps, where the blood supply is carried to the new site along with the flap tissue.

- **Full-thickness graft:** This refers to a graft composed of the donor skin's epidermis (outer or top layer) and the entire dermis (the layer below the epidermis that contains elastic fibers, connective tissue, hair follicles, nerves, and tiny blood vessels). The subcutaneous tissue, which contains fatty tissue, is not included. A full-thickness graft must be closed surgically.

- **Split-thickness graft:** This refers to a graft composed of the donor skin's epidermis and part of the underlying dermis. Thinner than a full-thickness graft, a split-thickness graft will heal on its own without being sutured onto the recipient site.

Definition of a Flap

In a flap, tissue is removed from one site and surgically repositioned to another location, carrying its blood supply along with it. In a flap, there must be at least one robust artery to supply blood to the site and several veins to allow blood to return back to the heart. A flap may consist of skin only, but it can be skin plus muscle and even bone. The blood supply is always carried with a free flap or pedicle flap.

- **Free flap:** In a free flap, tissue is moved from a donor site to a distant recipient site. Moving the tissue this far requires disconnecting the artery and vein completely from the donor site, then reconnecting the artery and vein at the recipient site. Making this reconnection of vessels to supply blood flow is done using microsurgical techniques. An example is the radial forearm flap (RFF), which will be explained below.

- **Pedicle or pedicled flap:** Tissue is relocated by way of a tissue bridge rather than isolated blood vessels. This does not require microsurgical joining of one blood vessel to another. (They are not separated, so they do not have to be reattached.) An example is the anterior lateral thigh flap phalloplasty (ALT), discussed below.

- **Delayed pedicle flap or delayed pedicled flap:** This refers to a flap where tissue is repositioned to cover a nearby site, leaving a "corner" or a bridge of adjoining tissue through which the blood vessels travel. This does not require microsurgical joining of one blood vessel to another. (They are not separated, so they do not have to be reattached.) In a delayed pedicle flap, the surgery requires multiple steps done at intervals of 1 to 3 months.

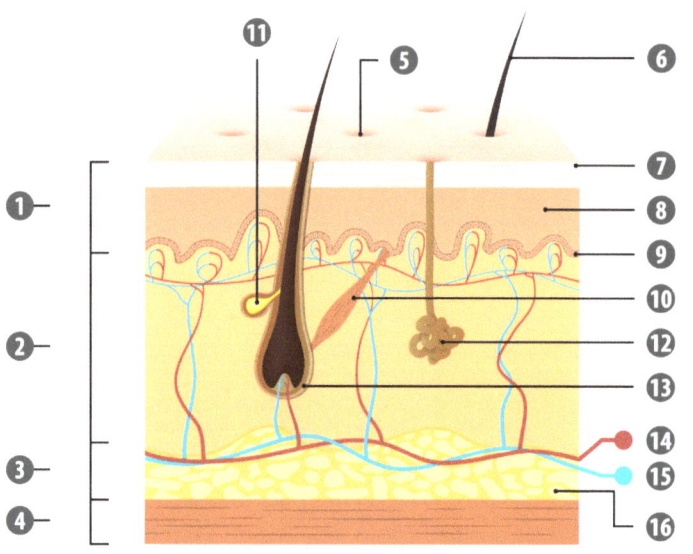

Figure 3.4. Structure of the skin.

Phalloplasty Options

The word *phalloplasty* is derived from the Greek and means "building a penis." Phalloplasty is much more complicated than metoidioplasty and its variations.

In practical terms, phalloplasty is far more expensive, more time-consuming (usually performed in several surgical procedures over 1 to 2 years), more difficult for a surgical team to perform, and more likely to have complications that will require surgical correction than other masculinizing genital surgeries.

All that said, phalloplasty creates a much larger penis, a penis that can penetrate a partner, and in many cases, a penis you can pee through. Here are the main categories of phalloplasty performed in the United States:

- **Radial forearm flap (RFF) phalloplasty**
  A free flap procedure where the neophallus is created from the radial forearm. (The radial forearm refers to the part of the forearm served by the radial nerves and blood vessels; "radial" refers to the radius bone on the thumb side of the wrist.) The forearm site is resurfaced by a split-thickness graft taken from the thigh.

- **Anterior lateral thigh (ALT) flap phalloplasty**
  The ALT phalloplasty is actually a pedicle flap phalloplasty where a flap from the thigh is carried by a bridge of tissue to form the neophallus. A split-thickness skin graft (also taken from the thigh) is used to resurface the ALT donor site. Donor tissue can also be taken from the side of the back using the latissimus dorsi muscle area. And there is another technique using the fibula (bone in the lateral lower leg) and nearby tissue. The latter two techniques are less common in the United States.

- **Delayed pedicle flap phalloplasty**
  In this technique, abdominal or groin tissue is used to create a nontubular (closed) cylinder, which is separated from its base at one end only. This creates a larger penis than with metoidioplasty. Penetration is possible with an implanted pump or malleable rod. A urethra may be reconstructed later and requires a microsurgical procedure. The delayed pedicle flap phalloplasty is done in several steps and is described on pages 84–87.

All Phalloplasties Require Several Steps

Most people coming to phalloplasty have already had a hysterectomy and bilateral salpingo-oophorectomy performed. As stated before, this is the removal of the uterus, cervix, ovaries, and fallopian tubes. A hysterectomy can be approached through a vaginal incision, a lower abdominal incision, or by way of robotic-assisted or laparoscopic techniques that add tiny incisions in the lower abdomen and belly button. If you have not had a hysterectomy done, you generally start with this. You may have a vaginectomy performed at the same time, but do talk to your surgeon about the technique and sequence they recommend.

In a vaginectomy, the vaginal lining tissue is removed so it can heal with one vaginal wall adhering to the opposite side. This causes the vagina to seal up and close the perineum so there will no longer be a vaginal opening at all. Particularly for nonbinary individuals, preservation of the vagina may be desired, along with creation of the phallus, although vaginectomy reduces the risk of fistula formation.

Please refer to these excellent medical illustrations done by artist Hillary Wilson. While the technique and the order of the steps may vary, these illustrations will give you a good idea of the basics of phalloplasty, complex as they are. Follow along with the illustrations as you read on.

Radial Forearm Flap Phalloplasty (RFF)

First Stage: Phallus Creation

- **The radial forearm site is prepared ("radial" means it is on the thumb side).**
  Generally using the patient's nondominant arm (that is, if you are right-handed, your left forearm will likely be used), the surgeon uses a template to trace the shape of the radial forearm flap. The flap is then surgically removed from the underlying tissue as a full-thickness flap, which includes the radial artery and veins as well as the lateral antebrachial sensory nerves and superficial veins. After this flap is removed, the donor site on the radial forearm will be resurfaced with a split-thickness skin graft harvested from the thigh.

  This patient will have already had electrolysis hair removal over the donor area. This is important, as the "tube in a tube" (which creates the penis) will have hair-bearing surfaces on the *outside* of the penis as well as on the *inside* of the urethra. The outside surface can be treated with electrolysis later if necessary. But hair on the *inside, lining the urethra itself*, is much harder to treat after the fact. (Allow 12 to 18 months for the electrolysis process to ensure adequate hair removal before phalloplasty.)

- **Removing the full-thickness radial forearm flap and then resurfacing the area with a split-thickness skin graft leaves a scar that closely resembles a burn scar.**
  Because this "forearm burn" is becoming so recognizable as a phalloplasty scar, some people worry that their scar may "out" them as transgender. Some men chose the ALT phalloplasty because the donor site scar on the thigh is more easily concealed by their clothing. (You may be able to minimize scarring with proper postoperative care of the donor site.)

  - **The new urethra is created by wrapping one side of the detached forearm flap around a urinary catheter.**

  - **The outside of the penis is created by then reversing the direction of the "wrap"** as the flap is wrapped the other way. Look very closely in the upper left portion of Wilson's illustration in Figure 3.5; you'll be able to appreciate this wrap and reverse-wrap.

Forearm Flap Phalloplasty Stage 1: Phallus creation

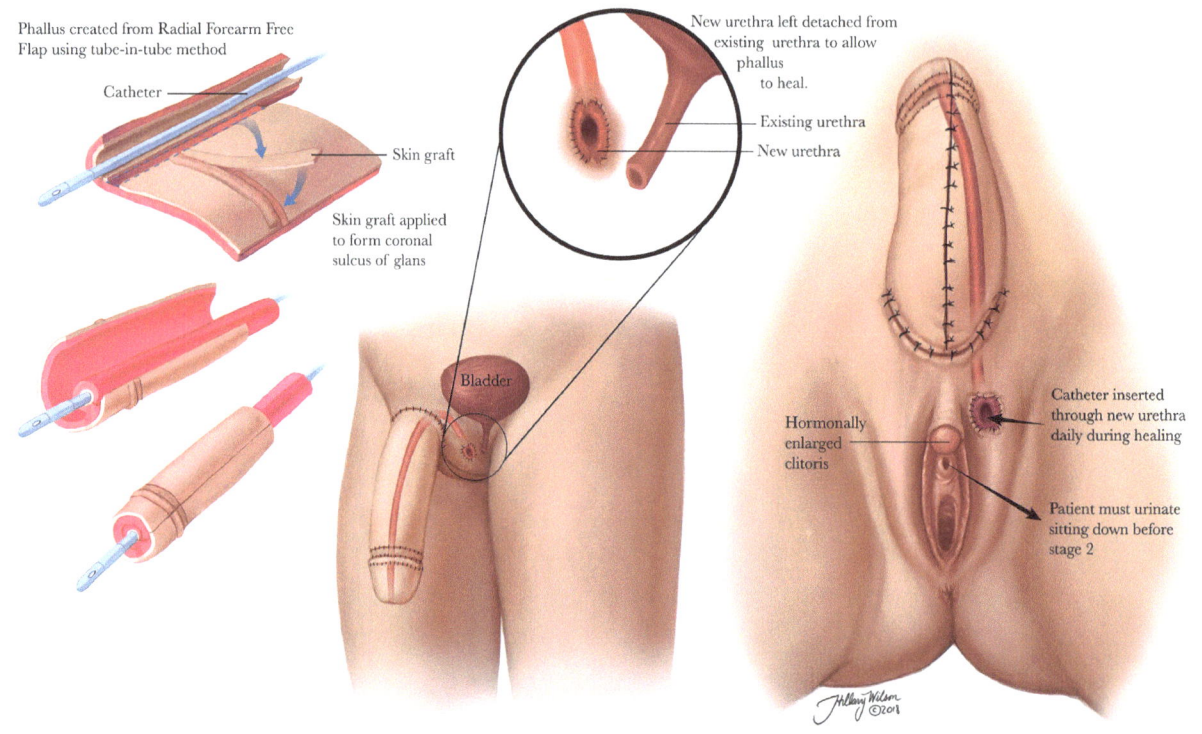

Figure 3.5. Forearm flap phalloplasty, Stage 1: phallus creation. Note in the upper left, the closeup of the neophallus creation from the radial forearm free flap using the tube-in-tube method.

Note also that different surgeons' techniques and sequences will vary. In the Wilson illustration, glansplasty is done at the initial surgery. Glansplasty is a plastic surgery technique. (One technique is to create two circumferential incisions parallel to each other at the end of the penis. The distal—more distant—incision is rolled under itself to create a "hem," creating the appearance of a circumcised penis (or the end of a noncircumcised penis with the foreskin drawn back.)

- **The end of the penis is sutured with delicate stitches to bring both layers of the "tube-in-a-tube" together.**
  This rounds out the end of the penis.

- **The neophallus is attached to the lower suprapubic area.**
  In the technique illustrated, the patient will pee sitting down through their original urethra for a while as the neourethra heals. Care is taken to keep the neourethra patent (unobstructed) by regular saline flushes (irrigations) through its catheter.

- **The free flap site at the radial forearm is covered by a split-thickness skin graft taken from the thigh.**
  This requires special care to facilitate healing: A wound VAC device or surgical compression bandages used for third-degree burns, and physical therapy are commonly used to protect mobility in the hand and wrist.

Second Stage: Urethral Lengthening and Scrotoplasty

Note: There is considerable variability from surgeon to surgeon. Some do vaginectomy in Stage 2. Some do glansplasty in Stage 2 or in a separate and brief outpatient surgery. Your surgeon will have their own reasons supporting their preferences for your surgery. Just be certain you know what you are having done.

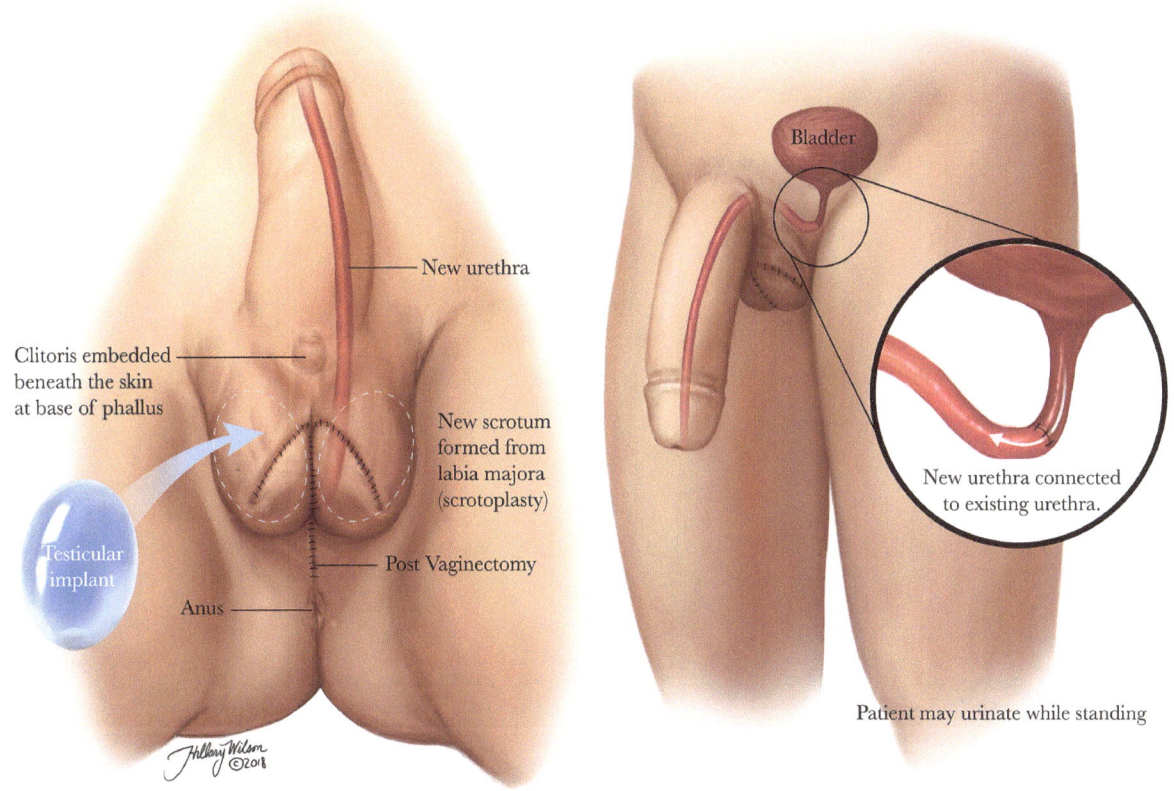

Figure 3.6. Forearm flap phalloplasty, Stage 2: urethal lengthening and scrotoplasty.

- **The clitoris is tucked under and *inside* the base of the penis, or it remains exposed and positioned *below* the base of the penis.**
  The nerves that serve the clitoris are then connected to nerves in the free flap. (More precisely, one of the dorsal nerves to the clitoris is preserved, and the other is connected to the nerves in the radial forearm flap.) This way, the primary erogenous sensation still originates in the clitoral tissue and orgasmic ability is maintained. Remember that the glans penis in phalloplasty will not have the same sensation as in a cis male; after all, the glans is newly constructed from the skin of the forearm (or the thigh in ALT phalloplasty).

- **A scrotoplasty is performed using the labia majora.**
  In Wilson's illustration, note the midline vaginectomy incision below the scrotum. Prosthetic testicles are placed in the scrotum, then or later. If more scrotal space is required to accommodate larger prostheses, tissue expanders might be placed first. The testicular prostheses replace the expanders later on.

As in anything in medicine or surgery, there is some controversy about the use of tissue expanders. Dr. Richard Santucci, citing the complications of eroded or infected scrotal tissue, stated, "I make the largest scrotum I can and at the 6-month mark, I can place bilateral testes implants…the weight of the scrotum acts as a sort of ersatz tissue expander."

- **The patient's original urethra is then connected to the neourethra.**
  If more urethral tissue is required, it may be grafted from buccal tissue in the mouth or from the free flap. The connection site, like anastomoses in general, may be the location of troubling complications such as urethral strictures or stenoses (narrowing), even to the point of obstruction. (**Note:** The terms "stricture" and "stenosis" are often used interchangeably.)

  If a stricture or stenosis occurs, the urine flow will slow down. It may require the use of a urethral dilator or a catheter on a temporary basis. In some cases, the urethra must be repaired surgically: "filleted" open at the site of the stricture, relined with buccal mucosa, and fully repaired 4 to 6 months later. The patient passes their urine through a suprapubic catheter in the abdomen as the urethra heals.

  Fistula formation, if it occurs, tends to happen at the "seam line" on the underside of the penis, particularly at the base or the tip of the penis. When a fistula forms, urine can leak out from the fistula as well as the opening at the end of the penis. These usually heal on their own but they can require surgical correction.

Third Stage: Erectile Implant

- **Erectile devices, such as an erectile pump or a malleable rod, are placed at least 8 to 12 months after the phalloplasty.**
  Initially, the new penis lacks sensation as the nerves are regenerating. What would happen if penetration was attempted too early with a pump or malleable rod in place? As the man pushed against a partner, the erectile device could poke through the penis! And the owner might not be able to feel it to recognize that this was happening.

  Wilson's illustration shows an inflatable erectile pump. Note that the pump device resembles a single corpus cavernosum. Also note the abdominal reservoir that holds saline before it is pumped into the device. And finally, notice the pump mechanism that is placed on one side of the scrotum. A prosthetic testis occupies the opposite side. Cis males with erectile dysfunction have used such devices for decades.

  While not illustrated, a malleable rod may be placed in the penis instead of a pump—again, after 8 or 9 months have passed. The rod can be moved from a downward position "at rest" to an upright position (or a 90-degree angle) for penetration.

Forearm Flap Phalloplasty Stage 3: Penile Prosthesis

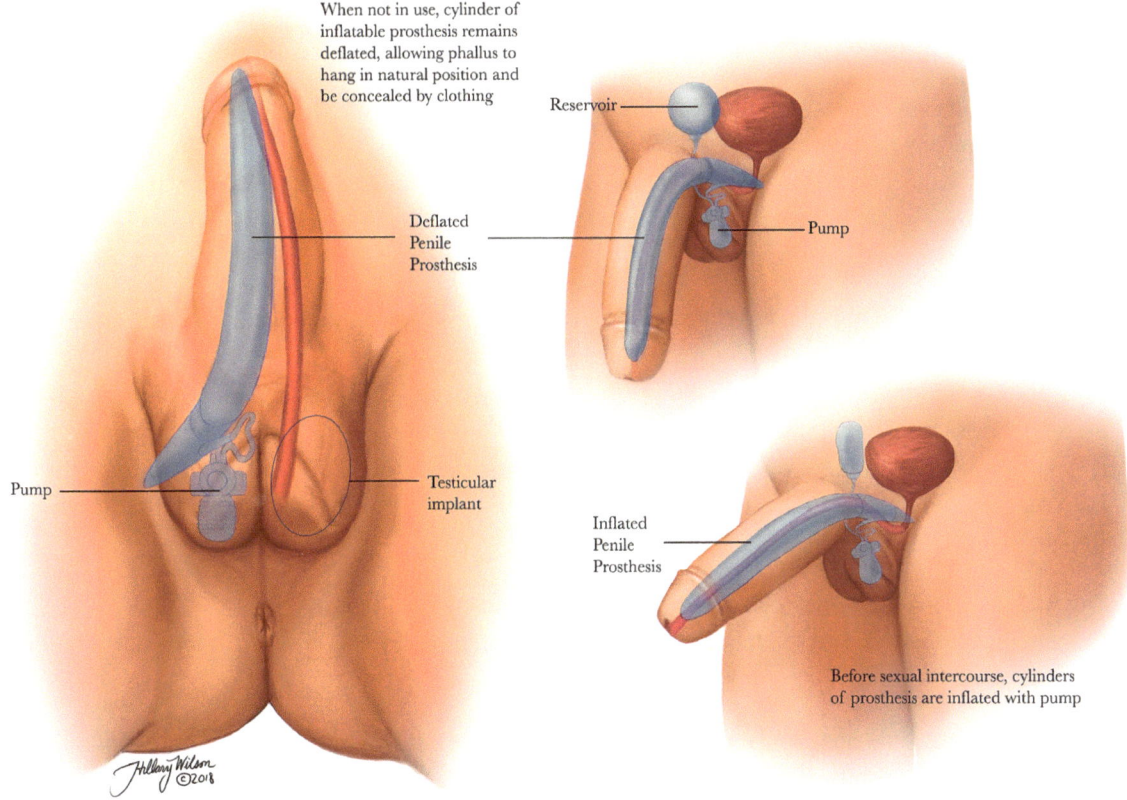

Figure 3.7. Forearm flap phalloplasty, Stage 3: penile prosthesis.

Shower or Grower?

A trans man with a phalloplasty is a ***shower, not a grower***! This expression means that the ***shower's*** penis size is the same whether it is flaccid (limp) or erect.

Many cis males experience enlargement of the penis as it becomes erect (they are ***growers***); the penis becomes longer and thicker. In a trans male, firmness occurs but growth in penile length and girth do not.

Anterior Lateral Thigh Flap Phalloplasty

- **The anterior lateral thigh flap site is prepared.**
  As before, electrolysis would have been completed, allowing 12 to 18 months for full clearing of the hair. A template is used to define the flap area and remove the flap from the donor location.

- **With its blood supply attached, the flap is moved under the groin muscles and through a groin incision to its anatomically correct position.**
  The ALT flap with its blood supply attached can be moved to a nearby location without interrupting its blood flow. The remaining steps are performed similarly to the techniques described in the part on radial forearm flap phalloplasty.

- **The skin of the ALT flap is thicker than a forearm flap, so it produces a penis that is very large (nearly the diameter of a soda can).**
  This phallus can be resized with liposuction later on, whereas the radial forearm flap is right-sized at its creation. Surgeon Richard Santucci points out, "A reality of ALT: If you have a thigh with a lot of fat, you will have a fat penis." Surgeon Toby Meltzer says, "An ALT flap is most suitable for a very lean male who has very thin skin over the thigh. Even then, it can be very large with a tube-in-a-tube design."

- **The ALT flap donor site must be covered with a split-thickness skin graft.**
  Care is similar with the ALT site, although mobility is much less of a concern than in the radial forearm, which requires physical therapy to ensure full wrist function later on.

- **If used as a shaft-only phalloplasty (no urethra), excellent results with normal girth and aesthetic appearance can be achieved.**

The Delayed Pedicle(d) Flap Phalloplasty (Also Called a Local Flap Phalloplasty)

A pedicle flap phalloplasty serves the needs of a trans man who wants a bulge in the crotch as well as the ability to penetrate a partner by way of an erectile device. In most cases, pedicle flaps are formed by creating a roll of tissue from the abdomen, thigh, or suprapubic area. The tissue roll will be relocated and reshaped over several surgeries, all the while maintaining the connection of the blood vessels at one end. The advantage here is excellent blood flow, and no microvascular surgery is required to connect donor blood vessels to recipient blood vessels. The blood vessels simply travel along in a bridge connected to the tissue.

> If you are preparing for a pedicle flap phalloplasty, exercise your whole body, but especially your gluteals, quads, hamstrings, back, and abdomen. This will help you develop collateral (extra) blood vessels. The better your blood supply, the better your pedicle flap will heal.

Although this type of phalloplasty is performed in several stages, each procedure is relatively short. This makes it a reasonable surgical plan for someone who is older or someone who may have more complicated underlying medical conditions and otherwise would not tolerate a lengthier time under anesthesia.

One of the most notable advantages of this technique is that there is no telltale graft scar on the forearm, so your business remains private. There is often significant incisional scarring at the donor sites, but these are easily concealed under clothing.

Let's look at an example of a delayed pedicle flap phalloplasty from the groin. When discussing pedicle flap phalloplasty from the groin, consider the following steps, which are completed over several months.

In each of the first four steps, you will note that the blood supply is maintained at one end of the solid tube created. Step 6 (glansplasty) and Step 7 (placement of erectile device) will occur 8 to 9 months later. Creation of a urethra can be performed, but it is a separate microsurgical procedure done later.

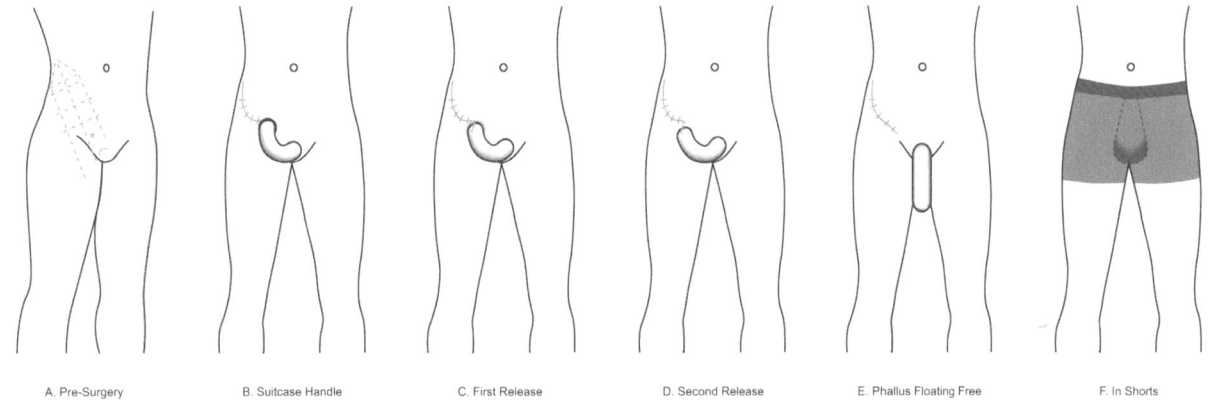

Figure 3.8. Delayed pedicle flap phalloplasty (glansplasty is not shown).

- **Step 1**

  The surgeon draws a template of the pedicle flap on the patient's body. In the groin technique, the flap is outlined with a surgical pen. The outline extends from the groin area all the way to the patient's back above the patient's waist. It is a larger, longer area than the size of the eventual penis.

- **Step 2**

  The surgeon cuts this skin and lifts it apart from the underlying tissue, leaving it attached at the hip end. It is rolled up into a tube, still attached at one end. The loose end (from the patient's back and waist) is rotated and reattached to the patient's midline (see Figure 3.8). When it is reattached, the closed cylinder looks something like an old suitcase handle. The donor site is sutured together, creating a linear scar on the side of the patient's hip and waist area. The patient stays in the hospital for 1 to 2 nights before discharge.

- **Step 3**

  At the next visit, perhaps 2 to 3 weeks later, the outside end of the suitcase handle is surgically narrowed by about 50 percent. The patient recovers with a tourniquet around the side that becomes the tip of the penis; he will gradually tighten this tourniquet per the surgeon's instructions.

  During this first delay, the major blood vessels that feed the flap are divided. The flap survives because of the new blood vessels that have formed at the base of the new penis and the skin that remains attached to the hip. As the phallus is fed by newly established blood vessels in addition to the original pedicle vessels, this tourniquet tightening will not compromise the overall blood supply. This process of delays allows the feeding vessels to be divided while the tourniquet stimulates increased blood supply to the entire flap. If the patient cannot use a tourniquet or cannot execute the process, a secondary additional delay can be done after the first one.

- **Step 4**

    About a month later, the lateral (hip side) attachment of the phallus is surgically narrowed again by another 50 percent. The patient again uses a tourniquet device, gradually tightening it over time according to the surgeon's instructions. As this surgical step is less complicated, the patient has this done as an outpatient procedure, not staying in the hospital overnight. The patient can also elect to have local anesthesia rather than general, if preferred.

- **Step 5**

    Several weeks later, the outer edge of the suitcase handle is completely divided at the hip and sutured closed. The flap is allowed to hang free, still attached with its intact blood supply at the patient's midline. The handle is then flipped upward (vertically) while still joined to the patient at the pubic area. The penis must remain in a vertical position for 3 months, again to maximize blood flow and to prevent swelling. The patient wears briefs or boxer briefs that secure the penis in the upright position.

    At each stage, nitroglycerine ointment is used to dilate surface blood vessels in another measure to ensure robust blood supply and flap survival.

- **Step 6**

    Glansplasty is the creation of a glans penis using a plastic surgery technique. These are done at many phases of a phalloplasty, from the initial surgery of the radial forearm or ALT phalloplasty to several months after the delayed pedicle flap phalloplasty.

    The timing is generally based on what has worked best for the surgeon in their experience. Some surgeons create two circumferential incisions and then "hem" the far incision to create the look of a seam. Others use a silicon cord to create a ridge that won't flatten out over time. Problems with the cord design include erosion and infection. Your surgeon is your best source of information, of course.

- **Step 7**

    If a man wishes to have an erectile device placed, this is done at a minimum of 8 to 9 months after the completion of the phalloplasty. This is to allow sensation to regenerate in the genital area so the man can have an erection and penetrate safely without the device poking through the side of his penis.

    The implantable pump erectile device consists of three parts. First, there is a tube that resembles a single corpora cavernosum, which is implanted in the center of the penis along its length. Then, a saline reservoir is placed in the abdomen to hold the saline to inflate the penile tube. Finally, a pump device is placed on one side of the scrotum (the scrotoplasty having been completed at an earlier surgery).

    The pump activates the saline reservoir to pour saline into the penile tube to make the tube firm. The pump mechanism also has a device to allow the penis to empty or relax after sexual activity by emptying the saline back into the reservoir. The owner pumps the device by squeezing it between the thumb and fingers.

A Surgeon's Advice

Due to its complexity from the sheer number of structures being created, as well as the requirement that they all work together in concert, phalloplasty remains one of the most challenging surgeries done in medicine. Along with this challenge come relatively high complication rates. By far, the most important step in the phalloplasty journey is preparation. Many patients end up with the feeling, "I never knew this could happen."

When considering phalloplasty, it will be important to arm yourself with the facts as best you can, and have those facts inform your expectations so that they are realistic. Speak with your surgeon carefully about all the techniques being used, design your particular surgery carefully depending on your desired functions, get a handle on the anticipated timeline, and make sure to ask not only about complications, but also how they will be managed and how they might change your timeline for recovery.

Just as in so many things with life, the goal in preparing for phalloplasty is to try and have no surprises. Be prepared for the worst and hopeful for the best.

— Dev Gurjala, MD

The following piece was written by UK blogger and vlogger Finlay Games. In this excerpt from May 25, 2019, Mr. Games writes about evaluating his own results.[26]

Managing the Expectations of Phalloplasty

Phalloplasty is all about managing expectations and getting to a place that's "good enough." Otherwise, we could spend our lives changing little bits here and there and never being happy. No penis is perfect. Penises come in all manner of different shapes and sizes and point in funny directions or have bends in them. As for phalloplasty, it's never going to be a cis penis no matter how many advancements the surgeons make. I believe that part of preparing for phalloplasty is acknowledging that fact and working out what "good enough" means for you.

For me, good enough meant being able to have a penis I could pee with and have penetrative sex with a partner. As long as it looked good enough to stand next to other guys at a urinal and make me smile when I looked in the mirror, that was good enough for me.

— Finlay Games

---

26   Finlay Games, "Phalloplasty Final Stage | AMS Implant Review," *Finn the InFinncible*, May 25, 2019, http://finlaygames.com/phalloplasty-final-stage-ams-implant-review.

Nonbinary (or Less Binary) Genital Surgeries

Penile Preservation Vaginoplasty with Peritoneal Pull-Through: Something New

> You will notice that I'm using the terms "penis" and "phallus" quite interchangeably. Embryologically, they are the same structure. Many nonbinary individuals prefer to use the more gender-neutral term "phallus" over the more male term "penis." Does it matter? It certainly can, so check with an individual as to what term they use.

The Penis/Phallus-Preserving Vaginoplasty with Peritoneal Pull-Through

Many transgender females who have both the funds and the opportunity choose not to have vaginoplasty at all. While many trans females are intensely dysphoric about even looking at their genitals, others prefer to keep the phallus.

I've begun to hear about a newer option for AMAB individuals who wish to preserve the phallus but create a vagina suitable for penetration—an adaptation of the vaginoplasty with peritoneal pull-through. (Refer to Dr. Wittenberg's information on peritoneal pull-through vaginoplasty on page 55.)

In this procedure or series of procedures, an individual first has an orchiectomy (removal of the testicles). A vaginal vault or cavity is developed starting from the perineum. A portion of the *peritoneum* is brought into the new cavity to line the walls of the neovagina. This *peritoneal* tissue is brought down from the abdomen by way of robotic-assisted laparoscopy.

(Refer to the "Perineum versus Peritoneum: Big Difference!" on page 55 to review the differences between the perineum and the peritoneum.)

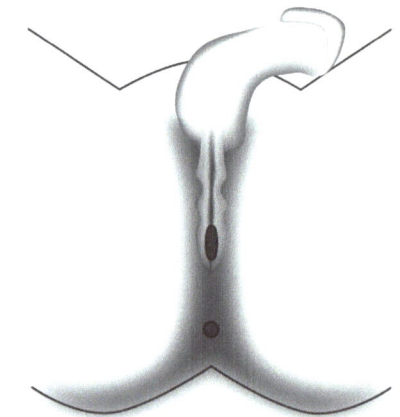

Figure 3.9. The penis/phallus-preserving vaginoplasty with peritoneal pull-through.

After a person has a phallus preservation vaginoplasty with peritoneal pull-through, the phallus remains above the opening of the neovagina. The phallus continues to serve as the main center for sexual pleasure and the conduit for urination.

The Penis/Phallus-Preserving Vaginoplasty with Full-Thickness Skin Graft

In the peritoneal pull-through procedure or series of procedures, the vaginal vault is developed in the perineum and lined with a portion of the *peritoneal* membrane that encloses the abdominal organs. This tissue is brought down from the abdomen by way of robotic-assisted laparoscopy. Here, the peritoneal membrane becomes the lining of the neovagina.

Alternatively, in the full-thickness skin graft technique, a graft is typically taken from the abdomen and is used as the lining for the vaginal canal. The skin graft is harvested using an abdominoplasty incision (a horizontal incision like you would see with a tummy tuck). The advantage of this approach, of course, is that you can get a tummy tuck at the same time. The disadvantage, when compared to the peritoneal-pull through, is the presence of a potentially long horizontal scar on the abdomen. Scrotal tissue is used to construct the labia.

The phallus remains above the opening of the neovagina. The phallus continues to serve as the main center for sexual pleasure and as the conduit for urination.

Seen on a social media site discussing penis preservation vaginoplasty:

Comment: "Yeah, but do you have a penis or a vagina?"

Response: "Yes."

Gender Nullification Surgery: "The Smoothie"

This procedure includes the removal of the penis and testicles and the reduction of the scrotal sac. It may also be referred to as the "Nullo." The urethra is shortened, so you pee through a urethral opening centered on the perineum but without a penis. The goal is to leave the area as a smooth, unbroken transition from the abdomen to the groin. Tissue from the tip of the penis can be buried under the mons (the lower part of the abdomen just under and above the pubic hair) for orgasmic response.

This surgery may be requested by people who identify as eunuchs and by others who wish an anatomically agender appearance. (See Davis Plastic Surgery's website at davisplasticsurgery.com.)

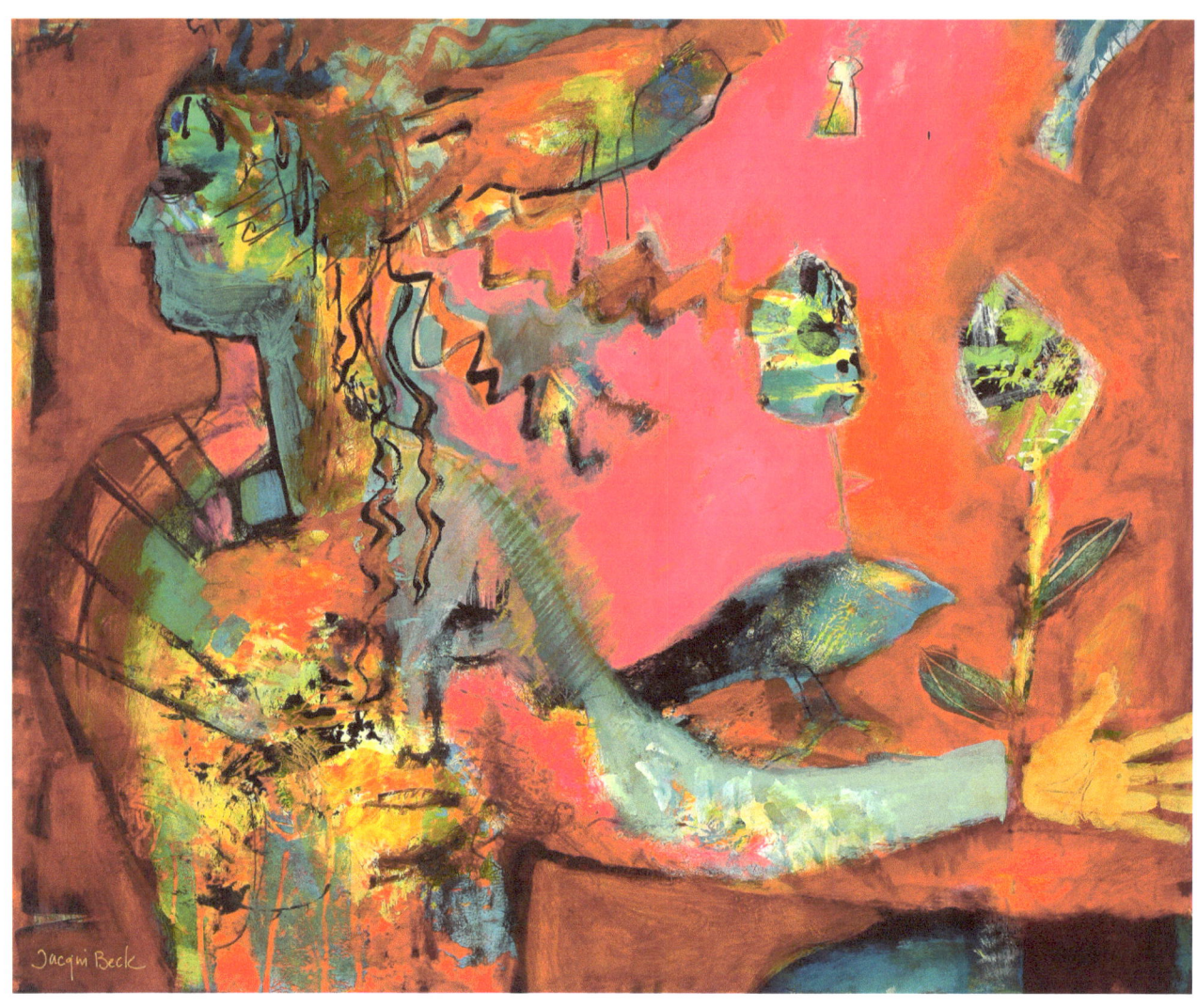

Inattention to Detail

CHAPTER 4
In Case of Emergencies

Recognizing When You Are in Trouble: Emergency Warnings That Apply to All Surgeries

We will address specific concerns relating to the individual surgeries later, but the following emergency information applies to all surgeries.

Post and Keep This Emergency Information on Your Phone

- Your surgeon's emergency contact number

- The address **where you are now**—that is, your own home address or the address of the place where you are staying

- Any personal emergency phone numbers, such as family and primary care physician numbers

Chances are excellent that you will get through your surgery and recovery with no major difficulties. But problems do happen, so it is important for you to know when to call for serious emergency help.

When to Call 911

- Call 911 if you are not getting enough air to breathe.

- Call 911 if you are having a severe allergic reaction (anaphylaxis).

- Your care partner calls 911 if you have passed out and cannot be revived.

- Your care partner calls 911 if you are not breathing and have no pulse.

- Call 911 if you are bleeding very heavily and cannot stop it.

- Call 911 for severe chest pain, "the worst headache of your life," seizure, severe injury, etc. If you think of calling, call.

Let's examine these in more detail. But stop reading right now if you are in the middle of any of these situations! **Call 911 and read later.**

- **Call 911 if you are not getting enough air to breathe.**
  - If you know you have asthma and are wheezing or coughing severely, use the asthma inhaler you have brought with you as you wait for the paramedics.
  - A pulmonary embolism (blood clot in the lung) can occur after a surgery. Symptoms can include shortness of breath, pain at the peak of each breath, upper abdominal pain, rapid or irregular heartbeat, coughing up blood, a swelling or lump in the leg, or dizziness, agitation, and loss of consciousness. If this is happening, you will need medical care in the ER.
  - There are other problems, such as panic attacks, heart rhythm problems, or even a heart attack, which can impair your breathing. Call for help.

- **Call 911 if you are having a severe allergic reaction (anaphylaxis).**
  - If you know you have severe, life-threatening allergic reactions called anaphylaxis, you will likely have your EpiPen with you. Use it according to the directions you've been given as you wait for the paramedics (remember that there are directions on the package). The paramedics usually carry EpiPens also.
  - Warning signs can include the throat tightness that comes from narrowing of the airway, hives, flushing, severe itching, and passing out.

- **Your care partner calls 911 if you have passed out and cannot be revived.**
  - Sit down, then lie down if you feel you are going to faint. It is always best to prevent fainting if you can.
  - If you have fainted quickly and without warning, you will likely regain consciousness rapidly as you are guided to a safe horizontal position. If you don't revive, your care partner must call 911 and follow the steps below.

- **Your care partner calls 911 if you are not breathing and have no pulse.**
  - If you are not breathing and have no pulse, your care partner must call 911 and start CPR (cardiopulmonary resuscitation).
  - The 911 dispatcher can talk a caller through CPR if they don't know how to perform it.
  - Continue CPR until the paramedics arrive and take over.

- **Call 911 if you are bleeding very heavily and cannot stop it.**
  - Apply firm pressure to the area of heavy bleeding.
  - As you wait for the paramedics to arrive, lie down with your legs elevated above the level of your heart (nipple level).
  - Call your surgeon as you are waiting for the paramedics. Your surgeon will help assess you and guide you further.

- **Call 911 for severe chest pain, "the worst headache of your life," seizure, severe injury, and other serious symptoms. If you think of calling, call.**
  - The paramedics evaluate a situation and provide emergency care. Many provide emergency-room– or intensive-care-unit–caliber treatment in the field. They will transfer a patient to the ER—or wait with the patient until a transport ambulance arrives.

Having an emergency like any of these by yourself emphasizes the need to have someone with you. But what if you are totally by yourself? In larger communities, dialing 911 (or even 9) will summon help. When you call 911, even if you cannot speak, dispatchers will see your address if you call from a landline. If you're using a cell phone, GPS tracks where you are located, but it can take additional time to locate you unless you've registered your address to connect it to your cell number. You also need to register your address to your phone number if you are using a voice-over-IP (VoIP) phone. Do the best you can in a situation like this.

What Happens If You Call 911 and It Turns Out to Be a False Alarm?

If the paramedics do not need to transfer you directly to a hospital, they will either call an ambulance for you or help you figure out what to do next (follow up with your surgeon, your PCP, and so on). They would much prefer to be called for a false alarm than to be called too late. If your situation improves markedly while the first responders are on the way, you can call again and cancel your request.

Other Urgent Situations You Might Encounter

The following situations require urgent attention but *may* not necessitate a 911 call:

You Are Suicidal

If you feel that you are unable to continue living and are thinking about ending your life right now, you must seek urgent help. This is a life-threatening emergency; the life that is threatened is yours! Depending on your circumstances, you must get yourself to someone who can evaluate and treat you. Naturally, you may certainly need to call 911.

You Are Having Pain

Surprisingly—and as callous as this may sound—pain may not represent an emergency. But it does need to be managed.

Important exceptions, of course, are chest pain or "the worst headache of your life," which may signal a heart attack or stroke, respectively. These circumstances definitely warrant a 911 call.

If you are having pain that is suddenly much more severe or different in character than the pain you have experienced, it is very reasonable to contact your surgical team and follow their guidance.

Remember also that regulations dealing with opiates have become quite strict. We cannot, for example, call prescriptions for narcotics into a pharmacy. Plan ahead and contact your surgeon's office before you run out of medications.

You Have a Fever

Take your temperature with the thermometer you were advised to buy before your surgery. A fever is technically defined as 100.4 degrees Fahrenheit, but use the guidelines your surgical team has given you. A fever may signal an infection, and you may need further care. (Sometimes, your temperature is elevated from atalectasis, which occurs when a person is not expanding their lungs enough with each breath. Many postoperative patients have to be reminded to take deep breaths or to use an incentive spirometer device from the hospital. But this problem is generally easy to solve.) Contact your surgeon's office and follow their guidance.

You Are Having Nausea, Vomiting, and Diarrhea and Are Feeling Progressively Weaker

While the reason for your symptoms may not be clear, you may need help to prevent further fluid loss. Of course, it is important to address the underlying cause of your symptoms. Contact your surgeon's office and follow their guidance.

You Are Having Urinary Symptoms

A burning sensation when you pee, peeing more frequently than normal, feeling the urgent need to pee and then peeing only a tiny amount, or peeing blood may signal infection. Or, if your urethra has been revised or built during your surgery and you cannot pee but your bladder is filling fast, you may have a blockage or narrowing (stenosis or stricture). No matter which problem you have, contact your surgeon's office and follow their guidance.

Lists like the one above cannot consider each and every problem that can occur after a surgery. Use your good judgment. Always remember that a call that turns out to be unnecessary is far better than a call that does not get made in a situation that turns out to be serious.

What happens if you cannot reach your surgical team? Contact your PCP, the emergency room, or the nearest urgent care center. It is fair to state that many ERs and urgent care centers may not have a great deal of experience with gender-affirming surgeries.

But do not delay the care that you need *now* based on prior experiences or fear.

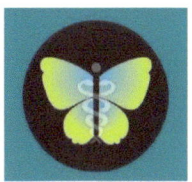

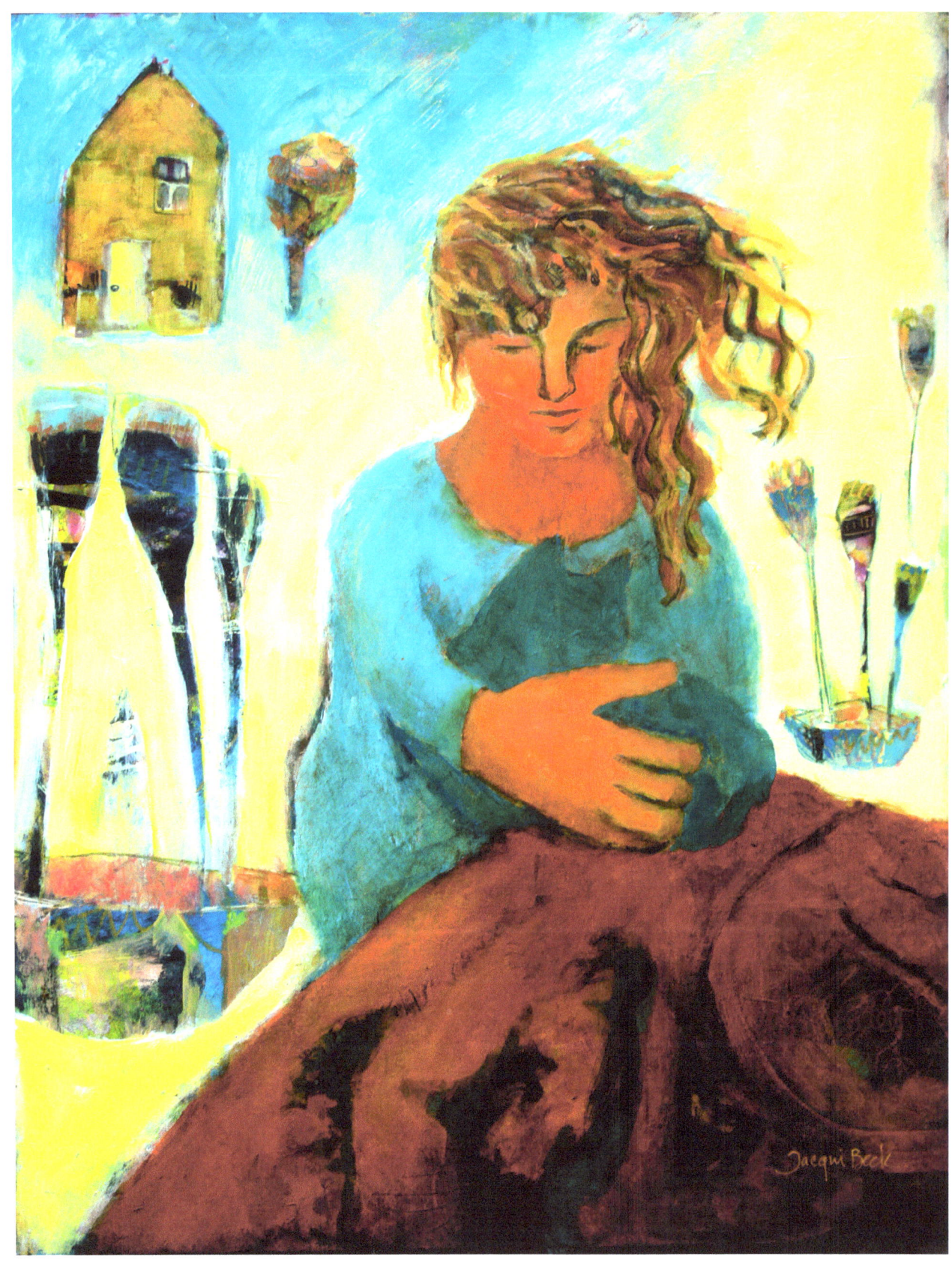

Comfort Found

CHAPTER 5
Taking Care of Yourself after Surgery

This chapter begins with what happens in the hospital and general postoperative principles that apply to all gender-related surgeries, followed by more specific recovery information for specific surgeries. It is important to keep in mind that everyone will have a unique postoperative course; no two people will have the same experiences.

As always, this information is intended to supplement information from your surgeon, not to replace it. If there is any disagreement between my information and that of your surgeon, go with your surgeon's recommendations.

What to Expect in the Hospital

Having a surgery of any kind can be intimidating, even overwhelming. I remember my family physician used to joke,

---

Q What's the difference between a major surgery and a minor surgery?

A A major surgery is any surgery done on my body. A minor surgery is any surgery done on someone else's body.

This probably rings true for all of us.

Let's begin by reviewing some concepts about surgery in general, regardless of which surgery a person is having. Most people undergoing a gender-related surgery are having an elective surgery. Does *elective* mean you don't really need it? Not in the least.

An elective surgery is *scheduled in advance* because it doesn't involve a medical emergency. (You could have an emergency gender-related surgery, of course, but that would likely involve an unexpected, rare complication that had to be handled urgently.)

A gender-related surgery usually has a time and a date planned ahead and is listed on a surgery schedule. It is usually performed during the day when the surgeon and crew are awake and everyone is fed and appropriately caffeinated.

You Will Likely Follow the Standard Routine

- Due to the coronavirus pandemic, you will be required to have a COVID-19 test to ensure that you are not infected before being admitted to the hospital. You must isolate yourself until the results confirm that your test is negative.

- You will enter the presurgery intake area, where your name and identity are confirmed. You'll be asked what surgery you are having and the name of your surgeon. A name band stating your name, birthdate, and likely your surgeon's name is fastened around your wrist.

- You will then go to a preanesthesia area where you dress privately in a patient gown, a paper shower cap, and nonskid slipper socks. A nurse or assistant again confirms who you are and what surgery you're having. They double-check that you signed your surgical consent (your permission to have the surgery performed) and that all of the required lab tests have been done.

- Next, you meet the anesthesiologist—a physician or a CRNA (certified registered nurse anesthetist). Expect to answer all the questions you've already been asked and to discuss more about your overall health, the medications you take, whether you've had anesthesia before, and whether you've had adverse reactions to anesthetics or allergic reactions to any medications. (If you find yourself annoyed by the repetitious questioning, remember that it is done as a double-check for your safety.)

- The anesthesia provider may examine your heart and lungs, and they may do an electrocardiogram (EKG). They assess your mouth, teeth, and airway to prepare to place an airway tube. (Even if they are not planning to insert an endotracheal tube, they assess your airway in case an emergency arises.) The anesthesia provider starts an IV to give you intravenous fluids and medications during your surgery.

- The anesthesia provider may give you a medication by IV to relax you before you're wheeled into the operating room (OR) on a gurney (stretcher).

If you're still awake as you are wheeled into the OR, you'll see many expensive machines all over the room. There'll be a scrub nurse dressed in a surgical gown, cap, gloves, and mask. The scrub nurse responds to directions from the surgeon and anticipates their needs, such as handing the surgeon instruments and suctioning blood away from the surgical site so the surgeon can see well. Also present is a circulating nurse, who wears scrubs, a mask, cap, and gloves. Because this nurse is not "sterile" like the gowned scrub nurse, they provide general support for the patient and everything that occurs in the OR, but they don't touch the site of the operation. ("Scrubs" refer to the loose-fitting clothing worn by many hospital staff. A scrub nurse is so named because they scrub their arms, hands, and fingernails prior to gowning up and having their gowns placed and tied.)

Your anesthesia provider stands or sits by your head, which will be at the head of the OR table; they monitor your heart rate and rhythm, your breathing rate, and your levels of oxygen and carbon dioxide as measured through a skin sensor. An anesthetic mask may be placed over your nose and mouth. If you're having general anesthesia through an endotracheal tube (ET) going down the throat, the ET is placed after you have been sedated by the IV medication. Your vital signs (blood pressure, pulse, oxygen level, and so on) are recorded continuously. If you're having a regional anesthetic, an epidural or spinal catheter is placed appropriately by the anesthesia provider. (The type of anesthesia given will have been discussed with you preoperatively.)

> In the OR, everything moves like a choreographed dance; everyone knows exactly what they are supposed to do. As a patient, gain reassurance from the fact that while this operation is new for you, it is very routine for your surgeon and the OR staff.

During your surgery, the surgeon, the surgical assistant, and all of the OR staff work together to accomplish the surgery that you have planned. If unexpected events occur, know that your team has seen such events before or have practiced ahead of time for nearly all possibilities.

After Surgery, You Will Be Moved into the Recovery Room or the Postanesthesia Recovery Area

In the recovery room, you will likely have one-on-one care by the recovery nurse until you are conscious and able to speak and swallow. Unless otherwise planned, your airway tube is removed, and you'll be breathing on your own without mechanical assistance.

Sometimes people go directly to their hospital room after surgery. In some cases (such as phalloplasties with microsurgical procedures), you may go directly to the special care or intensive care unit (ICU) for monitoring of your blood circulation at the microsurgical anastomoses of blood vessels.

If you end up being in the ICU but hadn't expected to go there, remember that the ICU affords you the most meticulous one-on-one care available. Sometimes a patient has experienced an unexpected event during surgery, such as an unpredicted fall in blood pressure, excessive bleeding, or an allergic reaction. In these cases, your surgical team has assessed that you need closer monitoring than the average patient and is moving you to the ICU for your safety.

When You Are Awake and Breathing without Assistance, You Usually Go to Your Regular Hospital Room

If you're having outpatient surgery (sometimes called a "day surgery" since you will be discharged home on the same day and not stay overnight in the hospital), you'll be observed in a recovery area until you're stable enough to have someone take you home. In general, your driver must be a partner, parent, or friend—not a driver for hire.

In your hospital room, your care is likely to be shared by several nurses and assistants. Depending on the size of the hospital, you will meet other personnel, such as laboratory technicians, physical and occupational therapists, social workers, dietary staff, cleaning personnel, pharmacy staff, and members of your surgical team, of course. Someone from the team (often a nurse practitioner or physician's assistant) will "round on you"—meaning evaluate you—at least daily.

In the hospital, expect to get out of bed with help and move around on the day of your surgery, or certainly by the next morning if your surgery is done late in the day. (This would not apply to patients who go to the ICU right after surgery.) Expect to be busy with wound care, bathing, resting, sleeping, eating, getting up to walk, discovering how to pee again if your surgery involved your urinary tract, and spending time with visitors. You may have to wait for various bodily processes (like bowel movements) to become automatic again. Some postoperative days will require more emotional energy than others.

You will likely have pain. Your surgical team expects this and will have provided orders for pain medication to keep you reasonably comfortable. Take your medications regularly; it's often easier to *keep up* with pain rather than try to *catch up* with it.

You may have a patient-controlled analgesia (PCA) device that allows you to get a safe dose of IV pain medication when you push a button. This allows you to get your medication without waiting for someone to administer it. However, the PCA device protects you from getting too much medication by having controlled dose parameters.

It's much more reasonable to anticipate having pain rather than expecting no pain at all. As you recover, your pain medication will come in pill form rather than via injection or through your IV. Many people require at least a limited supply of narcotics when they leave the hospital, although it is becoming increasingly common not to prescribe narcotics postoperatively. (Refer to the part on gabapentin and ibuprofen on pages 104–105.) Narcotics can constipate you, so drink fluids and take the fiber supplements and stool softeners offered.

The length of your hospital stay depends on the type of surgery you have had and the pace of your recovery. When you are ready for discharge to your home or a recovery facility, you will be given medications to take with you (and prescriptions if needed), written instructions on how to care for yourself, and information on where to call if you have questions or need immediate care. You will also be given information on when to follow up with your surgeon and your primary care provider (PCP).

General Postoperative Home Care Guidelines for *All* Surgeries

While every person and every surgical case is different, here are some general principles that apply to all surgeries.

You'll hear this qualifier repeatedly: If I present anything that conflicts with your surgeons' advice, listen to your surgeon and surgical team.

Your healing requires time, restorative rest, more protein than you might imagine, a healthy fluid intake, proper wound care, and gentle attention to your mental health. It also requires you to detect problems that do occur and respond appropriately so that you get the help you need. We will examine each of these areas and then go on to discuss considerations for specific surgeries in the parts that follow.

It Can Take a Village: Your Team of Support

Ideally, everyone undergoing any surgery would have a loving, nonintrusive guardian angel to welcome them home and then prepare food, help them bathe, fluff their pillows, change their surgical dressings, help them take their medications on schedule, drive them to appointments, and massage their shoulders. Sometimes, mothers who have just delivered a baby will hire a postpartum doula (a nonmedical support person) to help them when they first come home. I think everyone coming home from a gender-related surgery could use a doula and maybe such services will develop.

In fact, in researching this, I discovered a company of care providers who can be hired to assist folks after masculinizing surgeries when they stayed at the Quest House in Pacifica, California; visit t4tcaregiving.org for more information. See also the interview with the manager of Quest House on pages 135–138 on aftercare for masculinizing surgeries.

> Shortly before going to press, I learned that Quest House was closed due to lease- and pandemic-related problems. Then when making my final checks, I found that Quest House had reopened on a limited scale with expansion plans. Do check the website periodically to follow the progress of Quest House as the story develops (questhouseservices.wordpress.com).
>
> — Linda Gromko, MD

Care for patients undergoing both masculinizing and feminizing operations is also provided at the TransHeartline House in Marin, California (transheartline.org/services).

Perhaps you are fortunate enough to have a spouse or partner, a parent, a close friend, or a sibling to fill this role (or parts of it). Maybe you have the resources to hire a home health aide; if so, arrange this in advance and be certain that your assistant is trans-friendly and familiar with postoperative care.

Perhaps you want *nobody* around you as you recover. If that's the case, identify (and confirm) a few backup people you can contact if you do run into difficulties. If you live in an area where rideshare services are readily available and you can set up delivery services as needed, you will likely do fine for one of the less involved surgeries. But help can be wonderful, particularly in the postoperative period when you may feel more vulnerable than usual.

No matter what your circumstances are, you may find it helpful to go back and read Chapter 1 ("Planning for Your Surgery"). Also, review the checklists of helpful items to have on hand.

If you have a network of people like coworkers, friends, or a sports team, look at **Lotsa Helping Hands** (lotsahelpinghands.com) and **Meal Train** (mealtrain.com).

- **Lotsa Helping Hands** can help you or your point person organize people who want to be involved but don't know how to help you most effectively. If you anticipate needing extended support for making or providing meals, doing grocery runs, giving rides to doctor appointments, and so on, you can set up a free temporary website in advance to help coordinate the help you need.

- **Meal Train** is another web platform that helps you organize meals from your community of voluntary donors. Donors who couldn't (or shouldn't) spend time in the kitchen could opt to send a **GrubHub** gift card through Meal Train. Again, Meal Train is a free service, although coordinating additional services on Meal Train costs a small fee.

- **SignUpGenius** (signupgenius.com) is another group-organizing web platform you may like. It's free for friends and family to use.

- **Caring Bridge** (caringbridge.org) offers a different type of support. After you have a surgery, people will want to inquire on your well-being. You might find yourself facing a barrage of calls and messages at times when you're exhausted or simply need your privacy. Caring Bridge gives you a free web platform so you can issue bulletins to friends and welcome their support while maintaining personal boundaries. Caring Bridge asks for donations from readers, but it is quite unobtrusive.

Planning the Length of Your Recovery Time

For planning purposes, it's better to allow for a longer recovery period and be happily surprised than to imagine you'll be back in a few days and then find yourself tanking!

If you're having a major genital surgery, it is fully appropriate to plan for 6 to 8 weeks off work. Longer is certainly fine, depending on your situation. Some people plan for 12 weeks. You may be able to return earlier, particularly if you have the ability to start with part-time or to work from home. If you're having a less involved surgery, less recovery time will be needed. For example, breast augmentation would require less recovery time than a vaginoplasty. But add a few days of recovery time if you have *both* surgeries together. If you're able to return to work on a Thursday or Friday, or even go in every other day, do this to conserve your mental and physical energy.

Remember that recovery is not a linear process. I tell my patients to look at recovery as a spiral that gradually goes up: You progress a little, dip down a little, and spiral up again with the *net* direction in an upward progression. (But talk to your healthcare providers if your spiral moves perpetually downward!)

If you have to travel to a different city or country, allow additional time to recover from the travel itself. Often, the day you go home may take more physical and emotional energy than other days. Remember that the responsibilities that were shouldered by the hospital staff are now borne by you and your personal team.

Resting Effectively after Surgery

Your body needs rest and good sleep to heal. But surgery, anesthesia, pain, varying urinary signals, travel, and even your own excitement may disrupt your sleep patterns. Here are some considerations that may help you:

- **Relax your expectations.**
  It's understandable if you don't sleep perfectly after surgery. Most people don't! Try not to worry about not getting enough sleep. Set the stage to allow yourself to drift off to sleep. If you do sleep, fine. If you don't, just concentrate on resting and know that your body will still heal.

- **Create the most comfortable sleep environment possible.**
  If you can, clean your living space ahead of time so you come home to a reasonably orderly environment. Buy or borrow some extra sheets and pillows with pillowcases before your surgery. Use your extra pillows to help position your body to get yourself comfortable. For example, when you rest on your side, bolster your body with a pillow tucked behind your back, one between your elbows, and one between your knees, as shown in Figure 5.1. Or, get a body pillow.

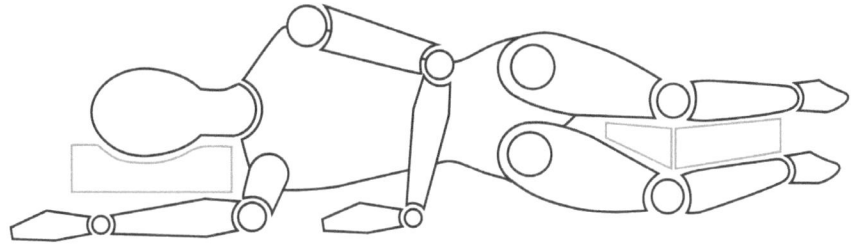

Figure 5.1. Resting on your side with extra pillow support.

If you have been advised to elevate your legs, it probably means elevating them above the level of your heart to help postsurgical swelling subside. A recliner helps, but you'll still need more elevation.

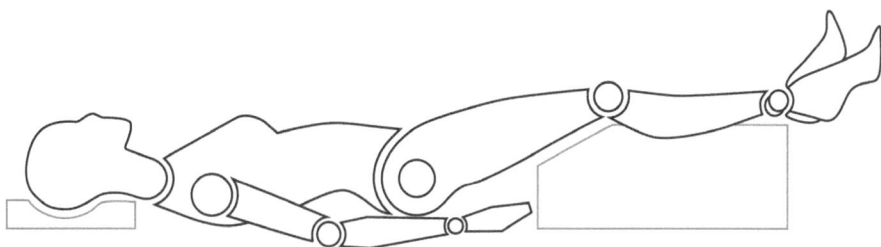

Figure 5.2. Elevation of the legs.

- **Stay clean and dry.**
  If you've had genital surgery, have some Chux pads, a waterproof crib liner, or even puppy training pads to place under your butt. These will keep your bed cleaner and drier and will be much more comfortable for you. You'll find a variety of sanitary pads to tuck into underpants or pajamas in the feminine hygiene or incontinence aisle of your grocery store, drugstore, or online retailer. (See the shopping list at the end of Chapter 1.)

  You may also appreciate having facial wipes and dry shampoo on hand if you cannot shower as often as you'd like. A hairbrush, a hand mirror, a tube of lip balm, and a container of simple lotion or moisturizer may help you feel better too.

- **Take a break from sleeping with your pets.**
  If you're in the habit of sleeping with your pets, take a break for 2 weeks to decrease your risk of post-op infections.

- **Keep some basic cleaning supplies near your bed.**
  You will appreciate having a box of facial tissue, a small wastebasket lined with a kitchen garbage bag, hand sanitizer, and a container of disinfectant wipes close at hand.

- **Set up your phone and charger.**
  For your comfort and safety, set up your phone and charger so you can reach them easily; buy an extra-long cord to make this convenient. It's never a bad idea to have a flashlight with you in case of a power outage. And you may need it for wound care anyway.

- **Create a relaxing environment.**
  A diffuser with essential oils provides relaxing ambience and makes your environment smell nicer. This may sound more like a frivolous luxury than a medical need, but feeling calm and breathing pleasant scents really can facilitate recovery. Unless you're allergic to essential oils, a small diffuser can bubble in the background, misting lavender or peppermint scents throughout your room.

- **Use white noise, ocean sounds, or quiet music to relax you.**
  If you have an electronic smart speaker, ask Alexa (or your Google friend) to play soothing sounds or music that you like, or wear noise-canceling headphones. Adjust your room temperature and lighting to make your environment more conducive to sleep. Consider getting a sleep mask to tune out ambient light. And then finally, just do the best you can. Even if you get sleep that's interrupted by pain, noise, or your bladder, it's better than no sleep at all!

- **Find a meditation app.**
  I first learned about the meditation-relaxation app Headspace from a client: headspace.com/headspace-meditation-app. She said that she never makes it to the end of a guided meditation—she's asleep by then! Headspace also tells you bedtime stories. (After a free trial, there is a yearly fee. But it's more cost-effective than a sleeping medication.) There are many similar apps. Here's a post that you may find useful: appsdose.com/2015/09/10-best-meditation-relaxation-apps-for-ipad-iphone.html.

Managing Postoperative Pain

Pain is expected after a surgery, although individual experiences vary greatly. Your surgical team expects that you will have pain and will give you prescriptions for medications to help you. Your medications may include any combination of the following:

- **Narcotics or opiates (although these have slightly different definitions, we will use the terms interchangeably here):**

  - Vicodin (hydrocodone + acetaminophen)

  - Percodan (oxycodone + aspirin)

  - Percocet (oxycodone + acetaminophen)

  - Dilaudid (hydromorphone)

  - Codeine

- **As you see from the list above, individual opiates may be prescribed by themselves or combined in a single tablet or capsule with ibuprofen (Motrin) or acetaminophen (Tylenol). These medications—**

  - Are *potentially addictive* but excellent for providing pain relief.

  - Are mind-altering—that is, they can make you "loopy"—and, if you combine them with anxiety medications or alcohol, you may get even loopier. It's best not to combine these without professional advice.

  - Have side effects such as nausea, vomiting, constipation, itching, and so on. *And you can be allergic to virtually any medication.*

- Are regulated with strict laws that govern the prescribing of such medications; we cannot phone these prescriptions into a pharmacy. Other people may steal your narcotics to use or sell. In our practice, we say, "If your cat eats it, your cat gets high." (No refills for meds that go down the sink, either.)

- Contain warnings like, "Do not drive or operate a forklift under the influence of these medications."

- Along those lines, make no truly important decisions while on narcotics. (As one physician friend advised, "Don't buy a grand piano while you're taking these drugs.")

- The effects of opiates can be immediately reversed by using the prescription medication Narcan (naloxone). If someone is living in your environment who is at risk for an opiate overdose, you may even want to consider having Narcan on-site.

Some surgeons are trying to eliminate the use of potentially addictive opiates in the post-op setting and are moving toward nonsteroidal anti-inflammatory medications and gabapentin.

- **Nonsteroidal anti-inflammatories (NSAIDs) (such as ibuprofen, naproxen, and aspirin)—**
    - Are available without a prescription; there are more potent ones that are prescription-only, such as ketorolac (Toradol). Do not combine prescription NSAIDs with over-the-counter NSAIDs as you can easily take too much.
    - Are not advised if you have an ulcer or kidney disease.
    - Have side effects, including gastrointestinal symptoms such as abdominal pain, heartburn, nausea, and vomiting. *And you can be allergic to virtually any medication.*

- **Acetaminophen (such as Tylenol)—**
    - Is generally well-tolerated and available without a prescription, but *you can be allergic to anything.*
    - Comes in a variety of over-the-counter mixtures designed to treat upper respiratory and sinus symptoms. If you are taking acetaminophen from several sources, be aware that it is possible to take too much! Add up the total amount of acetaminophen you are taking; generally, this should never exceed a total of 4 grams per day.
    - *Can cause liver failure with doses over a safe limit or intentional overdoses.* Check with your healthcare provider, your pharmacist, or even your local Poison Control Center if you're concerned.

- **Gabapentin (Neurontin)—**
    - Originally, gabapentin was used as an antiseizure medication; now it is mainly used for peripheral neuropathy and fibromyalgia, but it has been found to help with pain and anxiety. Dosages vary greatly; I start with low doses and increase gradually.

- Gabapentin is sedating at first before one adjusts to it; starting this medication at bedtime can help. If a person takes gabapentin for an extended time, tapering off it is done gradually to avoid precipitating a seizure or discontinuation symptoms (I hear patients complaining about "brain zaps" and anxiety if it is stopped abruptly).

• **Tramadol (Ultram)***

- Long described as a narcotic-like drug, tramadol is now considered a narcotic. This drug poses addiction risks and all the side effects seen with narcotics, such as constipation, sedation, and nausea.

*Note: Tramadol and Toradol sound a lot alike but are totally different medications with different side effect profiles. Know what you are taking!

Postoperative Nutrition: Getting Enough Protein for Wound Healing

You may not think of your surgical site as a wound. However, it *is* a surgically created wound and you must give your body enough protein to allow your tissues to knit together and heal. (When I see patients in my practice who are not healing quickly, we stress a jump in protein and fluid intake to accelerate a person's progress—and get some great results.)

Our primary nutrients consist of protein, carbohydrates, and fats. All are needed in the diet and all play important roles in tissue growth, maintenance, and repair. Most of us know about carbohydrates, which provide fuel for metabolic processes: sugar, flour, alcohol, and the complex carbohydrates found in starchy vegetables. Fats and oils (like butter, margarine, olive oil, lard, salad dressings) provide highly concentrated sources of calories, enhance the taste of foods, and are necessary for the integrity of cell membranes. Protein is made of amino acids that come from both animal and plant sources. Amino acids can combine to form the "complete" proteins that we do not make in our bodies.

Under normal circumstances, a person needs 0.8 grams of protein per kilogram of body weight. ***But it is estimated that a person healing from surgery needs 1.2 to 2 grams of protein per kilogram of body weight to heal well.***[27] But protein needs vary; a person with kidney disease may tolerate much less protein, while a person with a burn injury may require far *more* protein than usual after a surgery. If you have any doubt about your own situation, contact your healthcare provider and discuss this with them.

Here's how to do the math:

1. Figure out your weight: Take your weight in pounds and divide it by 2.2 to find your weight in kilograms.

2. Then, calculate how much protein you would need per day for postoperative healing (assuming that you do not require adjustments for kidney disease or burn injuries). Take your weight in kilograms and multiply by 1.2 grams of protein for the low end and 2.0 grams for the high end of the range of grams of protein needed per day.

Suppose you weigh 150 pounds (68 kilograms). You would need 54 grams of protein under normal circumstances (0.8 gram per kilogram of body weight) but you could need as much as 136 grams of protein per day for adequate wound healing. Tea and toast aren't going to cut it!

---

27   Chelsia Gillis and Paul E. Wischmeyer, "Preoperative Nutrition and the Elective Surgical Patient: Why, How and What?," *Anaesthesia* 74, Supplement 1 (January 2019): 27–35, https://doi.org/10.1111/anae.14506.

The point is clear: In most cases, you need more protein to heal well. Ask your surgical team or your primary care physician (PCP), or consult a dietitian if you have questions.

Protein Content of Various Foods from Animal and Plant Sources[28]			
Food (Animal Sources)	Grams of Protein per Serving	Food (Plant Sources)	Grams of Protein per Serving
Beef jerky (4 oz)	44 g	Soy protein powder (1 scoop)	20 g
Salmon (4 oz)	40 g	Veggie burger (1 patty)	12 g
Tuna (6-oz can)	39 g	Lentils or split peas (0.5 cup)	9 g
Steak (4 oz)	27 g	Edamame (0.5 cup)	8 g
Shrimp or prawns (4 oz)	24 g	Beans (kidney, garbanzo, navy, black, white, lima) (0.5 cup)	7 g
Chicken breast (4 oz)	23 g	Soy milk (1 cup)	7 g
Ground beef (4 oz)	20 g	Peanut butter (2 tablespoons)	7 g
Greek yogurt (8 oz)	22 g	Almond butter (2 tablespoons)	6 g
Cottage cheese (0.5 cup)	12 g	Whole-grain bread (1 slice)	4 g
Bacon (4 slices)	10 g	Steel-cut oatmeal, uncooked (0.25 cup)	4 g
Milk, whole (1 cup)	8 g	Hummus (0.25 cup)	4 g
Milk, nonfat (1 cup)	8 g	Brown rice (0.5 cup)	2 g
Milk, 2 percent (1 cup)	8 g	White rice (0.5 cup)	2 g
Egg (1 whole)	6 g	Almond milk (1 cup)	1 g

Table 5.1. Protein content of various foods from animal and plant sources.

If you are using prepared foods, read the nutrition labels to find out how much protein is contained in the food you eat. Pay attention to serving sizes so your calculations are correct.

---

28 Adapted from *Myfitnesspal*, v. 20.7.0.29453 (Under Armour, 2020).

Drink Your Protein

Protein Smoothie Recipe

1 banana, peeled
1 scoop protein powder of your choice (whey, soy, or pea protein)
¼ cup frozen fruit or frozen kale or spinach
5 to 6 ice cubes
2 cups water, milk, or milk substitute (almond, soy, cashew)

1. Combine the banana, protein powder, fruit or greens, and ice cubes in a blender capable of handling ice cubes (like a NutriBullet or Vitamix).
2. Pour in the liquid and blend away!

Iced Espresso Protein Drink

I wish I could take credit for this protein drink for coffee lovers. I've found it on multiple Pinterest and YouTube sites.

1. Buy a single or double espresso in a venti-size (24-ounce) cup filled with ice.
2. Pour an 11-ounce Premier Protein drink (try chocolate or caramel) over the ice.

This yields 30 grams of protein. Enjoy!

Getting Enough Fluid

How much fluid we need depends on our weight, our metabolic rate (the speed at which we use energy), our activity level, and the amount of fluid we lose through urine, blood, breathing, and so on. Tissue injury and wound healing also increase our fluid requirements. So does fever: We need more fluid to support the elevated heart rate and energy utilization we experience with fever.

At a minimum, plan on consuming at least 2 quarts of fluid per day as a baseline. A good rule of thumb is to drink until you have to pee every hour or two.

Volume Depletion and Dehydration: Not the Same Thing

Note that there is a difference between volume depletion and dehydration.

Volume depletion means that there is not enough fluid (blood) in the blood vessels, and **dehydration** refers to a lack of total body water.

For our purposes, we'll use the terms interchangeably, but it's not entirely correct.

While you're in the hospital, your surgeon and surgical staff keep track of your fluid balance. When you go home, you have to manage this yourself. Fortunately, our body gives us clues as to how much fluid we need. Here are some you may notice:

- **You're thirsty.**
  Thirst can be an indicator of decreased fluid volume; increase your fluid intake if you feel thirsty. Some people, particularly older people, may not be as sensitive to this indicator.[29]

- **Your urine is more concentrated.**
  Our urine gets more concentrated (darker yellow) when our bodies are trying to hold onto every drop of fluid volume. So, drink more fluid when you notice your urine looks more concentrated. If your urine is mixed with blood, it may be harder to see the color differences but do your best. (Brown urine that looks like cola can be a warning sign of an acute kidney injury; call your healthcare provider.)

- **Your urine volume is decreased.**
  If you are peeing very little, you may need more fluid. (This is different than not being *able* to pee—that is, having a full bladder but not being able to pass the urine out of your body. Contact your surgical team, especially if your surgery has involved reconstructing your urethra. You may have a blockage or narrowing of the urethra and need help quickly.)

- **You get dizzy and your heart beats faster when you first stand up.**
  When you first get up after a surgery, sit at the edge of the bed for a few moments before you stand. Then, get up carefully and make sure your body is steady before you walk. If you feel unsteady, sit or lie back down.

  Dizziness or rapid heart rate may signal low fluid volume. You can also get a low red-blood-cell count from blood loss, and you can have a rapid heart rate from fever. I might tell a patient, "Drink a glass of water or have a cup of soup. See if you feel any improvement over the next hour. If you don't, call your surgeon's office." (Call them regardless if you are worried.)

- **You are constipated.**
  Constipation can be a stressful problem after surgery. Opiate pain medications often slow bowel motility to a crawl. Then, if you have fluid depletion, your body tries to conserve every drop of fluid it can, even from the liquid stool moving through the large intestine. That makes the stool dryer and harder. Additionally, if you've had a genital surgery, you may not really *want* to push out a bowel movement because you fear that it may hurt. Make it easier on yourself by increasing your fluid and fiber intake and use laxatives, a laxative herbal tea (such as Smooth Move Tea), and the stool softeners that your surgical team recommends.

---

29   William Larry Kenney, and Percy Chiu, "Influence of Age on Thirst and Fluid Intake," *Medicine and Science in Sports and Exercise* 33, no. 9 (October 2001): 1524–32, https://doi.org/10.1097/00005768-200109000-00016.

Caring for Your Wounds

If you have a vaginoplasty, you will likely *not* have a postoperative bandage or dressing to go home with at all. You'll be wearing a sanitary pad in your underpants, and you'll change your pads, of course. But that's quite different from wound care after top surgery or donor site care after phalloplasty!

Caring for a postsurgical wound can be intimidating if wound care isn't in your skill set. It's all manageable, but it does take some attention to detail.

> Surgical instructions are not "guidelines" or "suggestions."
> They used to be called "orders." And they are there for your safety.

Before you leave the hospital, your surgical team will give you instructions on how to care for your surgical sites. They will show you how to change your dressings (bandages). Be sure you take any written instructions home with you, along with information on how to contact the surgeon's office for further troubleshooting. Follow your surgeon's instructions **to the letter**! Their instructions are provided for your safety.

Most surgical wounds *will* heal well provided that they are kept clean and dry and monitored carefully. Serious wound complications are rare, but they do happen. They can be treated, but occasionally some require a surgical revision. As stated earlier, you must support your body with plenty of rest, fluids, and excellent nutrition. Take the medications your surgical team has prescribed. Don't stop taking medications, particularly antibiotics, without your surgical team's okay.

> Our bodies are programmed to heal. When I was learning to deliver babies, one of my instructors said, "If you leave both halves of the vagina in the same room, it will heal."
>
> — *Linda Gromko, MD*

Changing Your Dressings: The Very Basics

STOP! Read this carefully.

Your surgeon will likely change your dressings the first time,
whether that is in the hospital or in their office.
Ask if you aren't certain.

If my comments are different than those of your surgical team,
follow their advice over mine!

The first few times you change a dressing, try to have another human with you for moral support and for more direct assistance. Put your animals in another room.

Review the following general principles *before you begin*:

1. Wash your hands with soap and water or rub your hands with hand sanitizer as instructed by your surgical team.

2. Assemble all of your wound care and dressing supplies before you take off the old bandages. Put your assembled supplies on an inexpensive flat tray that can be wiped down easily with an antiseptic wipe.

3. Set up your assembled supply tray in a clean area and on a clean surface. Be sure you set up the tray within your reach or within reach of the patient if you are the care partner.[30]

4. For wound care, you will likely use a mix of aseptic (very clean) techniques and a sterile technique. Your surgical team will help you figure out what parts of the dressing change can be aseptic and what *must* be sterile.

    - **Aseptic** (very clean) means devoid of bacteria, viruses, or fungi *that can cause disease*.

    - **Sterile** means devoid of *all* bacteria, virus particles, or fungi. This is the environment you want in an operating room. Do not touch anything that is supposed to remain sterile unless you are wearing sterile gloves and you understand sterile technique.

5. Tear or cut any tape you will need to secure the new dressing *before* you begin the dressing change. Many people place cut tape strips on the edge of their tray or table. The point is to have

---

[30] "Care partner" is the term that was liberally used in the kidney dialysis community in reference to the person who assisted a patient on home dialysis. I learned it from Dori Schatell, the executive director of Medical Education Institute, Inc.

your prepared tape ready and fastened to a place where you can reach it easily with a minimum of handling.

6. Set up a designated "dirty" wastebasket where you will dispose of the old dressings or other contaminated supplies. Line this wastebasket with a plastic kitchen garbage bag so it can be safely discarded separately from regular household garbage. You don't want kids or animals to get into this.

7. If you have Jackson-Pratt bulb drains to empty (the ones that look like small hand grenades), you may want to do this before removing the actual wound dressings. Write down the amount of drainage in each bulb. (This will help the surgical team estimate the proper time for them to remove the drains.) Wearing nonsterile exam gloves, carefully open the tab at the bottom of the bulb and empty the drainage into a designated "dirty" container. Recap the bulb. Cover the container and discard it in your "dirty" wastebasket.

8. Wearing nonsterile exam gloves, gently remove the old dressings. Discard the old dressings and the gloves you are wearing in the "dirty" wastebasket.

9. Take a careful look at the wound to assess the following:

    - **Redness:** Look for red streaks extending from the wound; notice any color you don't expect to see on a wound like gray or black.

    - **Swelling** of the wound and surrounding tissue.

    - **Pus or other drainage:** Clear serous fluid is straw-colored, while pus is white or yellow and has a thick consistency.

    - **Odor:** Notice if the wound has an odor, which can sometimes signify infection.

    If you see something that alarms you, have your care partner or assistant take a photo on a smartphone so you can share it with the surgical team.

10. Cleanse the wound as you've been instructed by your surgical team. Sometimes, you will do this in the shower right before you apply a new dressing; you may be advised to use a gentle soap and to allow water to run over the wound to rinse it. Or, you'll clean a wound using Betadine, provided that you are not allergic to iodine. You may be instructed to use normal saline to rinse the wound. (Saline is medically prepared, sterile saltwater.) Allow the wound to air-dry or gently pat dry with a sterile gauze square (which may be called a "four by four" because they measure 4 x 4 inches).

11. Wash your hands again or rub them with hand sanitizer. Put on the gloves as you've been instructed. These may be nonsterile exam gloves that come in a box or sterile, individually wrapped gloves like those used in surgery. Do what your surgical team has told you to do.

12. If you have been directed to apply any antiseptic or antibiotic ointment, gently spread it over the wound using a sterile swab or a sterile tongue blade. Start applying this at the area that must be kept cleanest (that is, the incision line) and work outward to the perimeter of the wound. This prevents moving bacteria into the area that must be kept the cleanest.

13. Gently cover the wound using sterile technique. Your team will tell you how to do this and what dressing material to use. If a wound is oozing, a layer of nonstick Telfa dressing may prevent the

wound from sticking to the bandages. Cover this with one or two layers of sterile dressings as you've been instructed. Cover this dressing with an outer dressing layer and secure this with the tape you have prepared. If you are using OPSITE (a clear transparent dressing that resembles a window), you won't need tape.

14. Discard used wound supplies safely in the "dirty" container, which is kept away from clean supplies, people and animals, and general household garbage. Any fluid or other material that drains from a wound is considered a biohazard and could potentially spread disease to another person. It is your responsibility to protect other people who could come into contact with biohazardous waste, so be sure to ask questions of your surgical team so you are comfortable with responsible biohazard disposal.

15. Recycle the clean wrappers from your dressing supplies. Use a recycle bin that is clearly distinguishable from your lined biohazard or "dirty" wastebasket.

If you require more complex wound care that requires assessment of other drains, or changing a wound VAC (vacuum-assisted closure) system, you will need more specific help. In some cases, you may be directed to go to a wound care clinic or your primary care provider's office. Or you may have a visiting nurse assigned to you. More information on wound VACs is on page 133.

Gentle Attention to Your Mental Health

The postoperative period can pose a significant disruption to a person's mental comfort. And why wouldn't it? You've just been through a major physical event that required years of planning and periods of logistical uncertainty. You may be under additional stress with travel, fatigue, medication side effects, and the need for more vigilance about your own health.

You undoubtedly have extra expenses, some of which you hadn't anticipated. You may feel isolated from people who ordinarily support you, such as coworkers and friends. You may have experienced worry or fear that you would not *survive* your surgery even though there was never any thought that your risks were excessive.

If you have a partner or spouse, you may find that your relationship with them has weathered stress too; some fundamental aspects of your life and relationship may have shifted. And if you do not have a significant other or supportive family members, you may feel more loneliness and vulnerability than you'd imagined.

If you've had a genital surgery, the world cannot possibly acknowledge what you've experienced. You have no cast or crutches that signal to others, "Please hold the door open," or "I could use help with this grocery bag." In fact, you may have just undergone one of the most significant events of your life and nobody really notices anything at all.

Answer this therapy question: **"If your best friend in the world felt exactly like you do now, what would you do for them?"** Have compassion for yourself and try to support yourself in the same way you'd imagine supporting a best friend.

Are You Depressed?

If you have experienced depression before, you may recognize some the following common symptoms:

- Sadness
- Feeling a sense of being let down or disappointed
- Fatigue
- Sleeping too much or too little; not feeling rested
- Crying more than you ordinarily cry, or not being able to cry
- Difficulty with focusing, concentrating, or reading
- Feeling irritable, cranky, or angry
- Feeling a lack of interest in things that ordinarily interest you or that you usually find pleasurable
- Feeling apathetic and not really caring about anything
- Eating "therapeutically"—that is, eating unhealthy junk food rather than healthy food that helps you heal
- Gaining or losing weight
- Experiencing excessive worry
- Feeling guilty
- Feeling isolated or that nobody really cares or understands

You may recognize that many of the above symptoms of depression actually overlap common postsurgical recovery experiences. If these symptoms are prolonged or severe, tell someone and get help. You may benefit from therapy or medications. Don't allow this to worsen.

As stated earlier in the pre-op part, if I know that a patient of mine struggles with depression, we may talk about starting medications *before* the surgery. Most antidepressants take 2 to 4 weeks to kick in.

> Be aware that you may be depressed and at serious risk if you're having passive thoughts about dying such as, "It wouldn't matter if I died," or if you're formulating a plan to die on purpose or by "accident."

Recognize That You Are at Risk

Tell someone right away so you can get help. Get evaluated promptly. Call 911, your local crisis clinic, or the Trans Lifeline—or go directly to your nearest hospital emergency room for a mental health assessment.

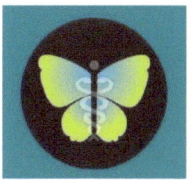

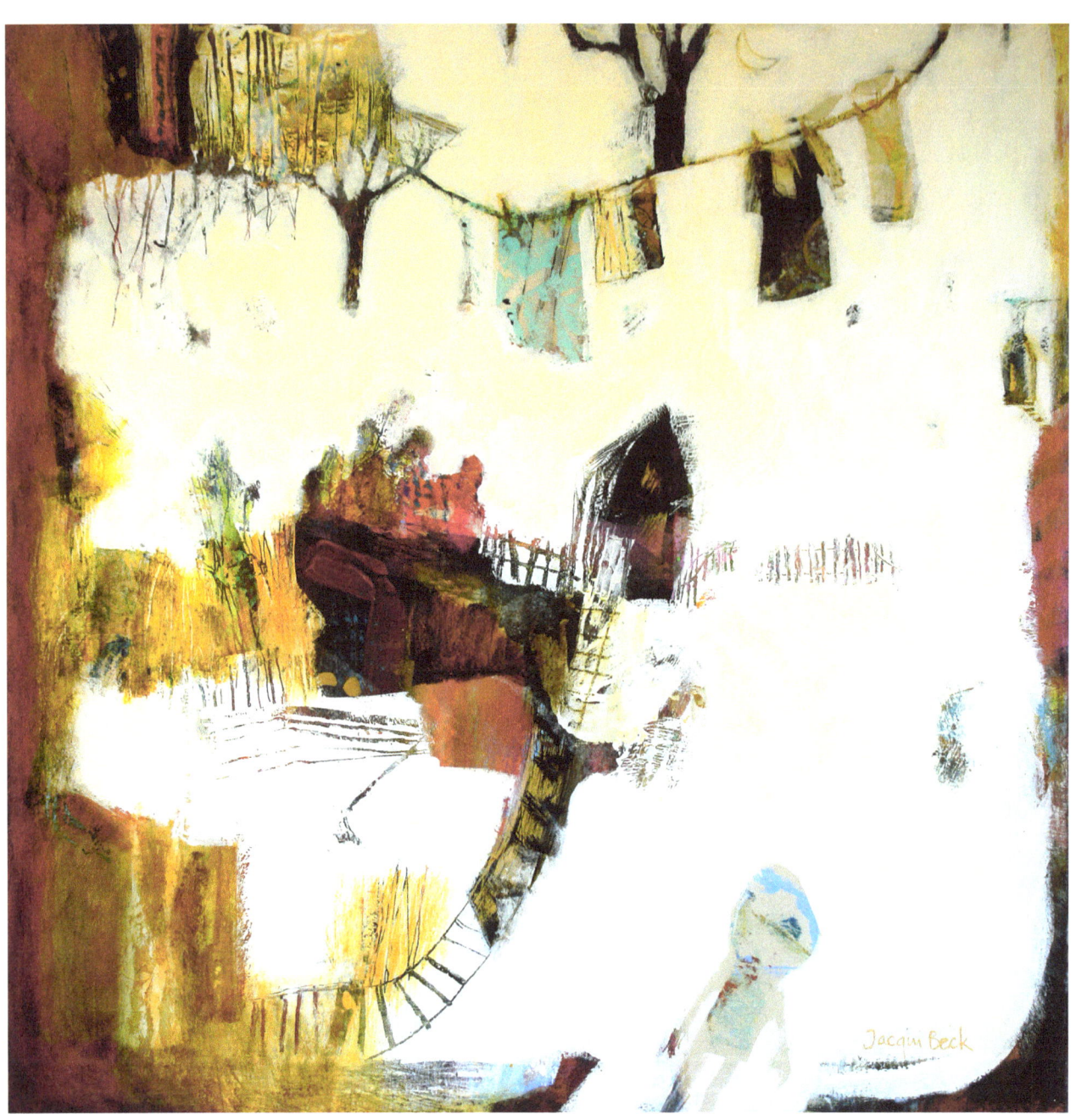

Feels Like Home

CHAPTER 6
Specific Postoperative Circumstances Dealing with Specific Surgeries

We'll address specific surgeries or categories of surgeries one by one and in the order in which they were originally presented. As always, your surgical team is your best source of information. Listen to them first!

Feminizing Surgeries

Facial Feminization Surgery: Post-Op Considerations

You may recall that facial feminization surgery (FFS) was referred to as a collection of surgeries done on the same operative day. The fact that it is a collection of several procedures may help to explain why most of *my* patients have found the immediate recovery period to be more difficult than with other surgeries they have had. That said, I know women who would disagree.

Here Are Some Pointers to Help You after Facial Feminization Surgery

- **Control swelling and pain with cooling and medication.**
  Swelling is intense, particularly in the early postoperative period. People may describe "bone pain" from incisions in the skull or jaw. Pain medication is prescribed, but ice packs may help also reduce both swelling and pain. The Facialteam (a facial reconstruction surgery group in Spain) uses "controlled cooling therapy" for the first 24 to 48 hours.

- **Eat well but gently.**
  Many surgeries are done through the mouth; in this case, you may feel like you have had a lot of dental work. Because you will need to eat plenty of protein to help your tissues knit together and heal, look for soft, protein-containing foods that don't require a lot of biting and chewing. You will be able to "gum" foods such as scrambled eggs, macaroni and cheese, and Greek yogurt. Liquid or semiliquid foods like protein smoothies and split pea or bean soups will be comfortable to sip.

  While not high in protein, Popsicles, frozen juice bars, or ice cream can soothe the inside of your mouth like an ice pack. Additionally, anything that is liquid at body temperature counts as a fluid. Fluid helps remove inflammatory debris and swelling.

- **Rest your eyes.**
  If your eyelids or the under-eye area are being modified, you may have swelling to the extent that it is difficult to see for a while. (Your eyes still function, of course, but it is impossible to see through eyelids that are swollen shut.) You may have extensive bruising and swelling. Here's where podcasts or audiobooks may help you get through!

> A 40-year-old woman told me after she healed from her FFS, "I looked in the mirror and said, '*There* you are!'" It was like she finally found the best friend she'd been looking for all her life.
>
> — *Linda Gromko, MD*

- **You may spit or vomit *some* blood.**
  If you have had a rhinoplasty (nose job), you may vomit some swallowed blood. This can panic you if you haven't heard of this before. Naturally, you should contact your surgeon if you're concerned.

- **Reassure yourself about your breathing.**
  Any swelling in the mouth, nose, or neck may make you feel like your airway isn't working properly. This may trigger feelings of anxiety or panic, such as feeling like you are not getting enough air to breathe. Sadly, we were all reminded during the George Floyd tragedy that a person may be able to utter sentences using very small amounts of air. So do not fall back on the old adage that "If you are talking, you are breathing." Try not to take on extra anxiety, which may only make everything worse, including pain.

- **Wear the compression garments that your surgical team advises.**
  Your surgeon is likely to have given you a snug facial or neck garment to wear as you heal. Follow your surgeon's instructions on how to use this correctly—that is, how often and for how many hours per day.

- **Gentle massage or manual lymphatic drainage reduces swelling.**
  You may be advised to massage parts of your face or neck. This is generally done to help mobilize the fluid that collects in tissues after surgery. Doing massage carefully will help the swelling go down more rapidly and you'll feel more comfortable faster. Your surgeon may advise you about manual lymphatic drainage (MLD). This is a very light-touch massage done to gently coax the lymphatic system to remove extra fluid and debris. Unless your surgeon advises otherwise, search the Internet for MLD therapists in your area.

- **Follow your surgical team's directions about physical activity.**
  The Facialteam notes, "Between 6 and 10 days after surgery, when acute inflammation and other symptoms are under control, the patient enters a 2- to 3-week period of progressive recovery, during which time we recommend minimal exertion. After this period, the patient can return to her usual routine. Moderate physical exercise can begin 3 to 6 months after surgery."[31] (Be sure your surgeon knows what kind of "moderate" physical exercise you do.)

Patience Is Critical!

It typically takes between 6 and 12 months to really appreciate the changes created by FFS. I usually tell my patients not to pass judgment until at least a year, but this is your face and it's visible to everyone!

As mentioned earlier, FFS is a surgery (or more accurately, a collection of surgeries) that can make the most impact reducing the effects of testosterone on your outward appearance.

---

[31] The Facialteam has a full playlist of videos that describe the process and many other aspects of facial feminization surgery on its YouTube channel: youtube.com/c/FacialteamEu/playlists.

A gentle reminder: ***Do not start smoking again after any surgery***. It's especially hard when you aren't feeling great and the full surgical results aren't visible. Do anything safe and legal to keep yourself from restarting.

Breast Augmentation Surgery

Follow your surgeon's advice to the letter. Read my guidelines about general surgical recovery. You will likely be able to go home on the day of your surgery unless the breast augmentation is combined with other surgeries such as vaginoplasty.

Be certain not to drive or use alcohol or other substances that make you drowsy while taking your pain medications. If you get into a crash, you could be cited as an impaired driver. Plus, you could hurt yourself or someone else.

In addition, you will want to clarify the following with your surgeon:

- When can you lie or sleep on your front or sides?

- What restrictions do you have on your body's movements? You may be advised not to raise your arms above the level of your shoulders for at least 2 weeks.

- When can you resume exercise? Be sure your surgeon knows exactly what type of exercise you are talking about!

- When can you buy new bras? Following surgery, you'll be required to wear a special postoperative bra except when bathing. (You will not wear new bras until your swelling decreases, likely at least 1 month postoperatively.)

- Will your surgeon (or their assistant) instruct you on how to perform breast massage to help the tissues heal (if that is required after your surgery)?

Orchiectomy

Orchiectomy, or the removal of the testicles from the scrotum, is generally an outpatient surgery (day surgery). It is helpful to rest, elevate the lower half of the body, and apply ice packs.

All postoperative guidelines apply here, but be sure to ask your surgeon and your PCP about stopping spironolactone or other testosterone blockers. Once the testes have been removed, these medications are generally stopped.

Vaginoplasty

Does My Vagina Look Normal?

One of the most common questions I hear from postoperative trans women is, *"Does my vagina look normal?"* And given the enormous variety among the genitals of all women, the answer is almost without exception, *"Yes!"*

The best illustration of this I know is a magnificent art piece titled *The Great Wall of Vagina*. British artist Jamie McCartney asked female volunteers to participate by making plaster casts of their labia! These casts were assembled in a collection of panels. In fact, it was one of my post-op trans women patients who first showed me this piece, which is Panel 4. The Great Wall can be seen in its entirety at jamiemccartney.com/portfolio/the-great-wall-of-vagina.

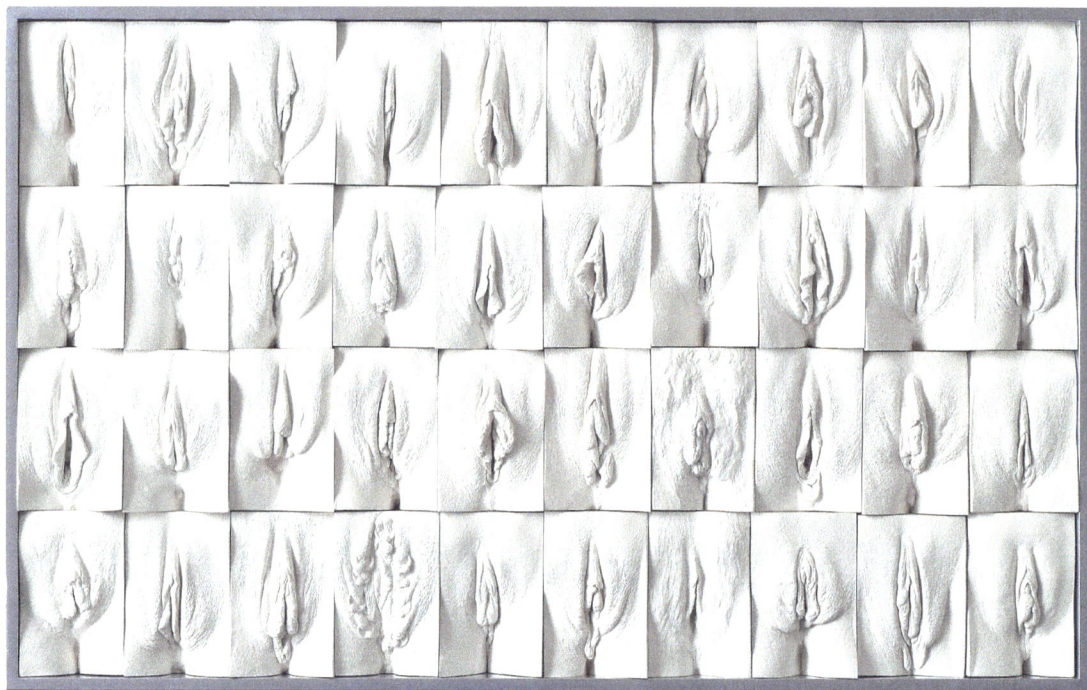

Figure 6.1. **The Great Wall of Vagina** *by Jamie McCartney.*

Another resource is *I'll Show You Mine*. This book, a photo collection edited by Wrenna Robertson, shows mostly cis women and some trans vulvas—each one unique. Reassuring and educational, many women don't have opportunities to view a lot of vulvas.

> As you are examining your postoperative genitalia, remember that you will "remodel" over time—even up to a year. Don't compare your early results with those of women on the Internet who have fully healed.

Dilation Is Critical

If you have a one-step or two-step vaginoplasty and you do not dilate, your new vagina can close!

I have seen this happen several times. It can occur in the span of only a few days, and it can be heartbreaking. It is possible that the neovagina can be revised and reopened, but this may require another surgery and such revisions are technically more difficult to perform. (It isn't known at this writing whether vaginal vaults created using peritoneal tissue require the same diligence in dilating. For now, follow your surgeon's instructions, of course.)

(This is where your pre-op planning is so important. If you really want to have only the phallus and scrotum removed but do not need to have a vagina that can be penetrated, consider a zero-depth vaginoplasty instead. The zero-depth vaginoplasty will take less surgical time to perform and require considerably less maintenance for you.)

Follow Your Surgeon's Dilation Instructions Precisely

You will have a dilation schedule to follow, as provided by your surgical team. As one example, you may be instructed to dilate three times a day for the first 6 months, twice a day for the next 3 months, once a day until the 1-year milestone, and weekly thereafter. But do not follow my schedule! Do what your surgical team has instructed. (Be sure to talk to your surgical team if you have had peritoneal pull-through surgery; those guidelines may be different.)

Surgical instructions are not "guidelines" or "suggestions"; they used to be called "orders" because the instructions are given to ensure that you have the best possible results and to keep you safe. So, follow these instructions even when you're tired and even if you don't want to!

Styles of dilation will vary from surgeon to surgeon. Some will have you insert your dilator to "depth" and stay there for 10 minutes or so; others feel that a rotatory or "dynamic" dilation is preferable.

Helpful Pointers for Dilation after Vaginoplasty

Dilating can be annoying and time-consuming. Many women feel that they've acquired a new part-time job after surgery. Here are some general guidelines for performing vaginal dilation:

- Wash and dry your dilator.

- Get all your dilation materials together before you start:

    - A towel or under-pad for under your butt

    - Surgical lubricant (water-based sterile lubricant like Surgilube, Slippery Stuff, McKesson)

    - A hand mirror and adequate lighting to see what you're doing (you won't need these for long)

    - Baby wipes, facial tissue, or a washcloth to wipe lubricant off your hands and clean up after dilating

    - Pillows and a blanket for comfort

    - Reading materials, TV, audiobooks, or podcasts at the ready

    - Any food or fluids you need for comfort and nutrition

    - Your smartphone to keep you sane, of course. But, if you see something that worries you about your healing perineum, take a picture with your phone and send it to the surgical team.

- Start with the smallest dilator to dilate, or the smallest dilator you used at your last dilation.

- Lubricate the dilator with sterile lubricant. In some situations, you may be advised to put about a teaspoon of medication on the tip of the dilator, so follow those directions if they apply.

    - Enter the vagina with the lubricated dilator, taking care not to touch or enter the urethra above or the rectum below the vaginal opening (women have dilated the urethra or the rectum by mistake).

- Apply slight pressure downward in the direction of the rectum as you enter the vagina; pushing up against the urethra may be painful.

- Take it slowly; don't force the dilator inside.

- Note the number of dots on your dilator once you have gradually reached "depth"—that is, the maximum depth you can comfortably reach or other depth measures you've been told about.

- Leave the dilator at depth for 10 minutes or the amount of time instructed by your surgeon. Some surgeons recommend a dynamic or rotatory process, so do this if instructed. Again, no freelancing.

- After completing dilation, clean yourself up with baby wipes or a warm soapy washcloth. Be sure to move front to back so as not to push rectal bacteria into your urethra, just as you wipe after peeing. Place a new sanitary pad or liner into the crotch of your underpants. At home, some women go without underwear in loose pants or a flowy skirt; tuck a washcloth in the crotch area in case you leak.

- Wash your dilator with soap and water. Then dry or air-dry it in a clean place so it's ready for the next dilation.

Dilation Q & A

Q Does having sex "count" for a dilation?

A No. Penetrative intercourse or penetrative sex toys should not be placed in the vagina by someone else for 3 months after surgery. For that matter, no internal speculum exams should be done for 3 months after surgery, unless approved by your surgeon.

Q So why can I dilate but can't have sex?

A When you are dilating, you know how deep you're going or if it is hurting or otherwise feeling different than usual. Somebody else cannot know this. Anal sex should not be practiced for the first 3 months also; the separation between the rectum and neovagina may be only millimeters in thickness, and anal penetration can cause injury.

Learning to Pee after Vaginoplasty

After vaginoplasty, you will have to get used to urination. Of course, you used to be able to aim your urine stream. After vaginoplasty, your urethra is much shorter, and the surrounding tissue will have varying degrees of swelling that will change from day to day. Your urine stream will run one way on one day and another way on the next! It may even spray like a shower head.

Here are some pointers to help you learn to pee again:

- This stream variation is temporary, but if it bothers you, consider buying a GoGirl, a Shewee, or other stand-to-pee (STP) device to guide the direction of your urine flow. Or try peeing through the core of an empty toilet paper roll or use a folded paper plate to deflect your urine stream.

- Gently wipe or pat yourself dry from front to back (from the urethra toward the rectum).

- If it is okay with the surgical team, you may use a peri bottle to gently rinse the perineum with warm water. Rinse from front to back and blot the area with toilet paper. A peri bottle is not to be inserted into the vagina.

- If you have been instructed to douche (that is, to rinse the inside of the vagina), follow the instructions from your surgical team. A douche has a rounded blunt tip, whereas a peri bottle has more of a point.

- Place a new sanitary pad or liner into the crotch of your underpants.

- Be aware of the signs and symptoms of urinary tract infections (UTIs); women get them more frequently because of the shorter length of the urethra and its proximity to the rectum.

Watch for the Following UTI Warnings

- Pain when you pee (during or as you finish); one of my patients described this as like "peeing pins."

- Frequency: peeing more often.

- Urgency: feeling the need to go to the bathroom right now.

- Peeing in very tiny amounts.

- Blood in the urine: This may represent a UTI, but it can also be associated with kidney infections, kidney stones, and so on.

- Fever may be associated with kidney infections and severe pain may occur with kidney stones; call your provider.

Swelling in the Perineum

Immediately after surgery, you may not be swollen at all. As you heal, the many incisions and tissue layers will draw fluid from your body into the surgical site. It is possible to have an accumulation of over a quart of fluid—although that is quite rare! Here are some tips to help you if swelling is a problem:

- **Moderate your activity.**
  Although you will want to be up and moving after surgery, too much walking may trap fluid in the perineal area. The same occurs if you are sitting in a "dependent position"—that is, your butt and feet are lower than your upper body and for too long a time. How long? Sadly, you must learn this from your own body; notice when your own swelling gets worse.

- **Elevate.**
  When you are resting, reading, or watching TV, try to keep your butt and legs elevated. Elevating above your heart level (nipple line) can be accomplished with pillows or foam wedges you can buy online.

- **Drink a lot of fluids.**
  This is so you mobilize the fluids retained in the perineal area. Watch your salt intake, as salt and water link together to hold excess fluid in your body.

- **Use ice.**
  An ice pack placed gently over the perineum may feel soothing and help reduce your swelling. You'll find a generous variety by searching "perineal" or "postpartum ice packs" online. A moldable bag of frozen peas is an old and less expensive stand-by that is flexible enough to fit the contours of your body. Wrap the bag first in a clean cloth or paper towel.

Constipation in the Postoperative Period

Narcotic (opiate) pain relievers slow the motility of your bowel. Take pain medications as directed but reduce your use when you can. Hydrocodone, oxycodone, and codeine can all constipate you—that is, make your bowel movements harder in consistency and more difficult to pass. You may not be eager to push anything out of your rectum since everything is tender. So, keep ahead of constipation by doing the following:

- Drinking a lot of fluid.

- Eating high-fiber foods.

- Trying a cup of Smooth Move tea or other laxative herbal tea. (Read the label, follow the directions, and don't try it if you're allergic.)

- Taking stool softeners and gentle laxatives (like Miralax) as directed.

If you go for more than a day or two without a bowel movement, increase your efforts to limit constipation. Call your healthcare provider if these measures don't work, especially if you've gone for 3 or 4 days without a bowel movement.

Common Worries

If Your Sutures Are Coming Out or the Incision Is Opening

It is normal for some sutures to dissolve and come out as you heal. Some sutures are engineered to dissolve while others must be removed; postvaginoplasty sutures are generally self-dissolving, for instance. Let these sutures come out on their own. Don't tug or pull on them.

Some wound separation is common with healing and usually requires no treatment. Talk to your surgical team and be prepared to send a photo taken with your smartphone if necessary.

If granulation tissue is identified (the pebbly, bright cherry-red tissue that you may see at an open incision line), your surgical team or other provider may treat this with silver nitrate. Silver nitrate sticks look something like long matchsticks. Once it is applied to granulation tissue, the silver nitrate helps heal the area and stops bleeding if it occurs. Expect a silver-gray discharge for a day or two after using.

Most of my patients have told me that silver nitrate is not particularly painful, although it is possible to have some temporary burning sensations with it.

If You Experience Vaginal Bleeding or See a Streak of Blood on your Dilator

Unless bleeding is profuse—in which case, call your surgical team right away—a small amount of persistent blood or a streak of blood on the dilator may indicate that you have an area of granulation tissue deep in the vagina or on a side wall. This can be treated with silver nitrate applications by your provider. As above, the silver nitrate chemically cauterizes the granulation tissue, reducing its size and tendency to bleed. It may take treatments on a weekly basis for a while (months in some cases), but it does heal. (No speculums for 90 days except by the surgeon!)

If you have not begun pelvic floor physical therapy, make these arrangements and begin now to maximize your urinary and sexual function.

Peritoneal Pull-Through Vaginoplasty and Phallus-Preserving Peritoneal Pull-Through

Many of the vaginoplasty guidelines—with the possible exception of the specifics of dilation—will apply. You will receive specific dilation information from your surgeon.

Have I forgotten anything? Quite possibly; everyone is different. Please call your surgical team if you experience anything that causes alarm.

Masculinizing Surgeries

We'll now address postoperative considerations in specific masculinizing surgeries or categories of surgeries one by one and in the order in which they were originally presented. As always, your surgical team is your best source of information. Listen to them first!

Remember that all of the same general postoperative information and warnings about dealing with emergent and serious problems apply.

Facial Masculinization Surgery

Facial masculinization surgery is a collection of surgeries that involve the bones and soft tissues of the face, scalp, and neck. Please refer to the postoperative recovery part for facial feminization surgery on pages 117–118. All of the concepts are the same or similar, although you may have an additional recovery area, such as the chest where the rib cartilage has been harvested. If you have had a rib harvested (or for that matter, any surgery involving the upper chest or collarbone area), it is possible—although unlikely—to experience the collapse of a lung due to even a tiny tear of the pleural membrane. This is treatable. Your surgeon will direct you to go to the emergency room if you are having difficulty breathing after your surgery.

After Gender-Affirming Chest Reconstruction (Top Surgery)

Nothing seems to impact the overall life experience of trans men like top surgery does. It is getting to be a commonly performed surgery that allows trans men to stop using the binders that have been so uncomfortable. It is frequently covered by insurance (sometimes even in adolescents). Nonetheless, it is a surgery.

Here are some points to consider to help in your recovery.

- *Do not start smoking again now* if you stopped smoking before your top surgery!
  Naturally, this would apply to any surgery. But it is critical in top surgery because the nipple is placed on the chest *as a graft*. Whether a graft "takes" or not depends on the blood supply at the surgical site. More specifically, this relies on the amount of blood delivered, the diameter of blood vessels, and the oxygen content of the blood. Smoking impacts all of these healing factors directly. You could actually lose a nipple graft if you start smoking.

- **Understand how much upper body movement is okay after your surgery.**
  I hear trans male patients referring to the "T-rex position" as a guideline for mobility after top surgery. The Tyrannosaurus rex was a dinosaur with tiny upper limbs that couldn't be raised even to shoulder level. Overhead stretching can disrupt your incision lines and increase your scarring, so move like a T-rex!

- **Expect to wear a postsurgical chest binder.**
  This binder is issued by your surgeon and may be even more restrictive than the binders you have worn in the past. It may zip together in the front or fasten together with hooks and eyes. Use this according to your surgical team's directions. This binder is temporary, though.

- **Sleep on your back.**
  Ask your surgical team about when you may sleep on your sides or front. Pillows or body pillows can help you.

- **Ask your surgical team about scar care.**
  Scars are raised and red for about a year, at which point they tend to become less visible. You may also notice a numbness around the periphery of the scars; this is also normal and will resolve in about a year also.

- **Consider using Pink Pockets to help you if you have post-op drains.**
  The mother of one of our patients is a nurse practitioner in the breast oncology department of a major medical center. She told us about Pink Pockets, a remarkable and inexpensive invention that allows you to secure post-op drains to your shirt, thereby reducing the amount of tug on the drains. They are pink out of respect for folks after breast cancer surgery, but they work for anyone who has a bulb drain after surgery. Search for **pink-pockets.com.**

- **Talk with your surgical team about nipple tattooing if, after about a year, you are still having hypopigmentation (reduced pigmentation) over the areolas.**
  The Vinnie Myers Team creates 3D areolar and nipple tattoos that are extremely realistic. One of the cisgender breast cancer patients in my practice had their tattoos by the Team after breast reconstruction. She was ecstatic about her incredible results, and I was simply astonished. I spoke with a representative of the Team, and they do nipple and areolar tattoos on trans men as well. This could include 3D tattooing if your nipple graft didn't "take" well. Contact their office via the website at vinniemyersteam.com to get an appointment in the Maryland studio and to learn the Team's travel itinerary.

  If you search the Internet for "nipple tattoos for trans men," you will find others across the country. (Refer also to the phallus tattoos on page 134.)

- **Don't burn your binders. Launder and donate them!**
  Imagine how much another transmasculine individual might appreciate inheriting your gently used chest binders! If you don't have a personal friend who would benefit, consider donating them to one of the many organizations that distribute used binders to trans men coming along the path. Point of Pride is one such organization; research them at pointofpride.org/donate-a-binder.

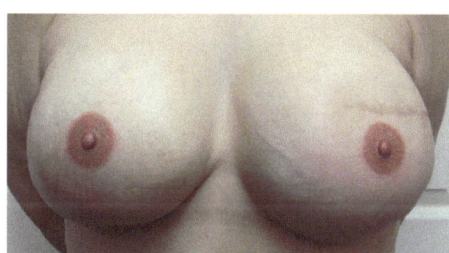

Figure 6.2. A 3D nipple tattoo done on a woman after a breast reconstruction surgery. While these nipples look like they protrude, they are absolutely flat to the touch. The Vinnie Myers Team, who did this tattoo, also does 3D tattoos for individuals after top surgery as well as penile tattoos.

After Hysterectomy and Bilateral Salpingo-Oophorectomy

Many—but not all trans men—have their uterus, fallopian tubes, and ovaries removed. Certainly, it is done in preparation for phalloplasty. Removal accomplishes the following:

- It essentially eliminates the possibility of cancer of the uterus, cervix, ovaries, or fallopian tubes. (Fallopian tube cancer is quite rare, but it can occur in people who have BRCA1, BRCA2, or other gene mutations that also increase the risk of a person getting breast, ovarian, peritoneal, fallopian, or pancreatic cancer.) Typically, cancers of the ovary, fallopian tubes, or peritoneum have subtle symptoms that are recognized late in the disease process. Particularly for trans men who are reluctant to seek out gynecological care, removing these organs can be smart.

As a reminder, top surgery does *not* eliminate the possibility of breast cancer, so chest exams done by a man and his healthcare provider are important. The evaluation of any lump is critical, as is special attention to those men with cancer-provoking gene mutations as mentioned above.

- Removal essentially eliminates the possibility of vaginal bleeding that comes from the uterus, which may occur when people run out of their testosterone, forget to take it, or are prescribed a dose that is too low. Bleeding can also occur because of a disease state, such as cancer. That's why bleeding that *doesn't* correct with hormone adjustments must be evaluated further.

Hysterectomy and bilateral salpingo-oophorectomy can be combined with procedures that reduce incontinence of urine or stool. This can be an issue for trans men who have had vaginal deliveries before transition.

Hysterectomy and bilateral salpingo-oophorectomy can be accomplished through the abdomen or through the vagina. But today, these procedures are often done using minimally invasive surgical techniques, such as laparoscopic and robot-assisted procedures. These enable the surgeon to make much smaller incisions. The organs are clearly seen when a camera (the laparoscope) is placed through the belly button, and photographs are projected on large screens opposite the surgeon and assistant. In robotic surgeries, the surgeon actually manipulates the "hands" of the robot and the camera remotely via a computer.

If you have a laparoscopic surgery performed, carbon dioxide gas will flow into your abdomen through the camera port to distend or raise your abdominal wall and make your organs more visible. Visibility is critical for precision! The CO_2 gas floats upward toward your diaphragm (the muscle that separates the abdomen from the chest). This in turn may cause you to experience "referred pain"—in this case, pain that originates below the waist but registers in the upper back or shoulders. Pain in these locations can understandably worry a patient who has had a pelvic surgery, but it is common and it resolves as the body eventually absorbs the gas.

A hysterectomy used to require 6 days in the hospital and 6 weeks off work, but minimally invasive techniques have generally changed all that. Today, it is usually an outpatient surgery (also called day surgery or ambulatory surgery), although some people stay for overnight or for a day or two.

After Monsplasty

Again, your recovery will depend on what technique was used. I had one patient who required a drain with a lengthy horizontal incision across the lower abdomen (although this is rarely needed). This foot-long plastic ribbon sat at the base of the surgical wound, exiting from one side. The ribbon had holes along it to collect fluid and worked something like a drain. Your surgical team or primary care provider can remove this under the surgeon's direction. (I appreciate that many people worry about how it will feel to have a drain removed, but most people don't have these drains at all.)

To remove a drain, I snip the sutures that are securing it. Then I ask the patient if they're ready and then instruct them to breathe in as I count to three and to blow out when I reach "3." When the patient is exhaling, I pull the drain out. The whole thing takes 30 seconds, the patient is distracted, and we're done, with "no trauma, no drama."

After Vaginectomy

In vaginectomy, the walls of the vagina are essentially closed together, which eliminates what some people refer to as the "front hole." It is frequently done in combination with other surgeries, and the postoperative vaginoplasty course may be dictated more by what else has been done as opposed to the vaginectomy alone. Expect pain and swelling, both of which can be managed by following the surgical team's directions.

> If you have a urinary catheter, your surgical team will teach you how to manage it. Although you will not have to *change* your own catheter, you will have to empty the urine bag. Sometimes patients are told to remove their own urinary catheters when they no longer need them. (You don't just tug or pull on it; you must first deflate a small balloon that holds the catheter in your bladder. If you need to do this, your surgical team will instruct you.) You should also know how to flush (irrigate) the tubing with normal saline to keep the urine flowing freely into the bag.

After Metoidioplasty

As with vaginectomy, metoidioplasty may be combined with other surgeries; your recovery course may be dictated by the associated surgeries. If you have had a metoidioplasty by itself, your recovery will be limited to the area of what used to be called the clitoris, which now becomes the neophallus. You will not be able to pee through the neophallus unless you have had a urethral extension.

Expect swelling in the area. The swelling may change from day to day, and it may be significant enough to impact your urination, but you should still be able to pee. While it sounds counterintuitive, drink more fluids so you make more urine. This will accomplish a couple of things:

- It will make you feel the need to pee more clearly, and the urine will typically come out faster with more volume and pressure behind it.
- It will make your urine less concentrated. Concentrated urine might irritate the sutures and sensitive surrounding tissues.

Although the swelling will go down in time, you can help reduce it and relieve pain by using ice packs. You can find form-fitting ones online (try searching "perineal surgery ice packs," but I found a much better selection by shopping under "postpartum ice packs"). I know that this reference may trigger dysphoria, but you may appreciate anything that works if you truly need this product.

After Metoidioplasty with Urethral Extension (Lengthening)

Metoidioplasty with urethral extension is naturally more complicated than metoidioplasty alone. Any time that you have your urethra lengthened, there is a risk for narrowing at the connection, which can slow or even stop your urine flow. Your surgical team will tell you what to look for, but here are some things to know:

- You will likely get donor tissue for your urethral extension from the buccal mucosa (the inside of your cheek), from the inside of your lower lip, or from the vaginal labia. These areas may hurt also. Your surgical team will give you tips on how to manage this pain.

- You will have a catheter in the neourethra for several weeks as it is healing. But your urine will actually be emptied through a suprapubic catheter in your bladder; it protrudes from your lower abdomen above your pubic bone.

After Scrotoplasty with Prosthetic Testes Placed

Like all tissue in the perineum, the new scrotum can accumulate fluid after surgery. Expect swelling. A scrotum can easily accommodate a liter of fluid. Reread the part on general postoperative care. For scrotoplasty, you will want to keep your perineum elevated when you are resting. This helps to reduce the amount of fluid the scrotum collects.

You may notice that the testicles are uneven in their location, or that one "rides up." Your surgical team will instruct you on how to massage your testicles so they stay down in the scrotum more easily.

If you have tissue expanders, you will be given special instructions on how to care for them. They will need to be filled periodically with normal saline; like many medical procedures, it isn't that difficult but requires careful attention to what you are doing.

After Phalloplasty (Free Forearm Flap and Anterior Lateral Thigh Flap)

As the most complicated of all gender-affirming surgeries, phalloplasty must be regarded as a combination of surgeries done at different times and with different purposes. Remember that the overarching goals of phalloplasty are to create the following:

- A phallus that can be used for urination, with the man standing up and urinating through his phallus.

- A phallus that can be used for the sexual penetration of a partner.

- Intact orgasmic function.

- Intact urinary function.

- Removal of the uterus, fallopian tubes, and ovaries (hysterectomy and bilateral salpingo-oophorectomy) is usually done early in the sequence. A vaginectomy is also recommended as it is associated with less fistula formation. A fistula is a hole that forms where it doesn't belong; it this case, it can cause leakage from the phallus in phalloplasty. They often heal on their own, but it's better not to get one!

The following information is designed to assist you in your surgeries and recoveries. Since there cannot be a single document suitable for each person going though these surgeries, do read widely, talk to your friends who have had similar surgeries, trust your surgical team, and ask a lot of questions.

This website also has some good information: healthcare.utah.edu/transgender-health/gender-affirmation-surgery/phalloplasty-recovery.php. **If there is a single matter of primary importance in phalloplasty, it has to be the blood flow to the neophallus.**

If you have had a microsurgical connection of a graft or grafts, you may spend your first few days in the intensive care unit or in a special care unit where you are monitored every 1 to 2 hours. This will vary from surgeon to surgeon and facility to facility. If you do go to a special unit, here's what you can expect:

- Your vascular connections where blood flows between a flap or graft and the neophallus will be monitored using a Doppler ultrasound device that attaches near the blood vessel connections in the penis. Other factors like color, warmth, and capillary refill will also be frequently assessed.

- You will be on at bed rest for most of the initial recovery and likely will have SCDs (sequential compression devices) that are wrapped around your legs to periodically squeeze them to move your blood along. This reduces the risk of blood clot formation, as does the use of anticoagulants.

- You will have a urinary catheter in your bladder, but it is inserted in the lower abdomen above your pubic bone. Your urine will empty through the suprapubic catheter (not through your penis) for the first few weeks. You will be trained in how to empty your urine bag and take care of the catheter. You will have another catheter in your penis to keep the neourethra open. This catheter will be removed around your fifth postoperative day, before you leave the hospital. And sometimes, men will leave the hospital with the urinary catheter in place and have it removed in the clinic later.

- You will have a PCA (patient-controlled analgesia) device during the first day or two after your phalloplasty to help you manage pain. You will also receive antinausea medication to keep you from vomiting, thereby keeping your body more stationary.

- You can expect to hear monitors and see LED indicators of various vital signs and body functions if you are in the intensive care unit (ICU). Your sleep will be interrupted, and you may require medications to help you relax and sleep. The sensory overload that occurs in the ICU can make you feel disoriented and you may appreciate medication for anxiety during this time.

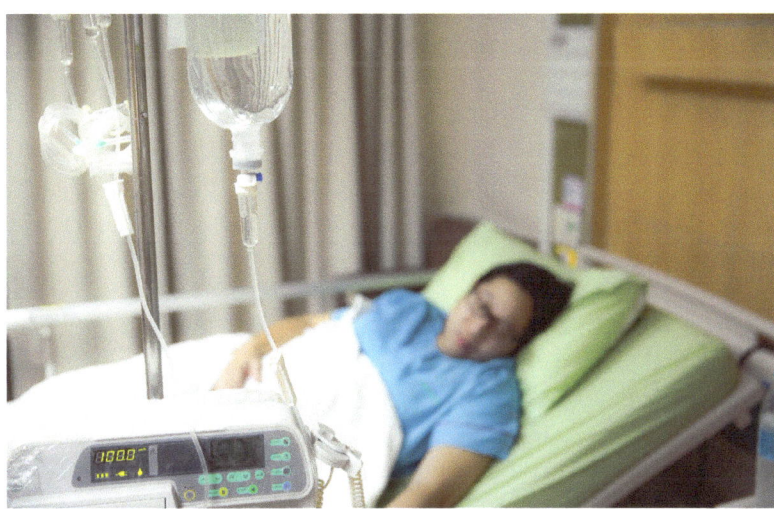

- You will receive fluids and some calories through your IV during your first 24 hours. You may not take anything by mouth in case you have to go back to the operating room quickly (usually to correct a blood flow problem).

- You will likely be moved to a less intensively monitored hospital room on or about the second or third postoperative day.

- Your penis will be elevated in a specialized dressing, and you will continue to be monitored closely.

- You will likely be up and walking and taking all your food, fluids, and pain medications by mouth on about the fifth day. You may be ready to be discharged.

- You will be given detailed instructions on how to take care of your skin graft site.

- You may expect to do physical therapy to keep your wrist, hands, and fingers supple if the donor site was your forearm. You may require a hand therapist, who is a physical therapist who specializes in hand rehabilitation.

- You may receive a specialized burn bandage to help your forearm heal.

- You will be taught how to take care of your penis and how to change your dressings.

- You will be taught by your surgical team how to elevate the penis and how to move your hips, legs, and the rest of your body to ensure adequate blood flow to your penis.

- You and your home caregiver must know how to care for any surgical drains you have. This will not be difficult, but it can feel that way at first.

You will be ready to leave the hospital on or around the fifth day postphalloplasty, provided that you are eating, taking oral fluids and pain medications, and that you do not have obvious problems that need to be addressed.

Problems at this stage include infection, bleeding, inadequate blood supply to the penis or graft sites, the inability to walk without assistance, or the inability to eat and take pain medications by mouth.

Before you leave the hospital, review with your surgical team the care of your penis, your donor graft site, your urinary catheter, your drains, and your surgical dressings. Make certain that your care partner has also received all their instructions. Also make certain that you have the surgical team's contact information available so that the team can "talk you down from the tower"—that is, help you problem-solve a difficult or puzzling situation if needed.

You will be required to stay within a 3-hour radius of your hospital for a couple weeks to a month after the surgery. If you live nearby, you can go home. But if you don't live nearby, you may stay with family in the area. Or you will have made reservations at a hotel or a recovery house well before your surgery. (See the information on Quest House on pages 135–138.)

After phalloplasty, you will be **expected and required** to have a care partner who will help you when you are discharged from the hospital. This can be a life partner, friend, family member, or someone you hire specifically for this purpose. This individual need not be a medical professional, but they must be precise in following directions, as they will be helping you with your dressings, your medications, and your general care. They must see *you* as their priority. (They cannot see you as their ticket for a vacation.)

If you are interested in hiring someone for this purpose, ask your surgical team for recommendations or search online. *Get references.*

Review your postoperative care supplies and make sure that you have everything that was recommended. You can still order things online if needed. A comprehensive list from Meiko Xavier is found at this website: myphalloplasty.wordpress.com/2016/09/28/medical-supplies-packing-list.

With the bulk of your surgery completed, don't let down your guard about your good self-care.

Follow postoperative pointers that are both general and specific to your surgery. Review the importance of getting sleep, consuming good nutrition, and keeping your mind sane. **Whatever you do, do not start smoking. The health of your blood vessels is critical to your healing.**

What Is a Wound VAC?

You've already read that having a wound VAC (vacuum-assisted closure) would elevate you to a more sophisticated level of wound care (see page 80). A wound VAC is an ingenious device that allows you to place a spongy material over the wound and cover this with a special plastic wrap and a dressing that attaches to a portable suction. This facilitates the continual removal of debris and drainage and greatly decreases the amount of time required for healing.

Urinary Leakage after Phalloplasty

> The best product I've found for leaking at the tip of the penis is the Male Urine Guard by Jackson Medical. They say it holds up to 2 ounces of urine—so it works great for "dribbling."
>
> — *Trans man, age 62*

After a Delayed Pedicle Flap Phalloplasty

The pedicle flap phalloplasty is done in several stages, and each part of the procedure requires its own specific recovery time. Your surgeon may have different requirements for each step.

Remember that the blood flow to the developing phallus requires the utmost protection. Check the temperature of the skin of the phallus. If it feels cool (as in cold) or appears dusky or pale, this may mean that the blood supply has been compromised. Contact your surgeon. They will have instructions for you and may require you to be evaluated in person.

Report any signs of infection (pus, inflammation, tenderness, fever, or general worsening) to your surgical team.

> I had had a metoidioplasty and urethral extension before. I've just had a pedicle flap phalloplasty. I'm so glad I did this. Now I look down and see my penis. There's nothing to put on and I don't have to worry about anything falling off. As far as urinating goes, I pee through the metoidioplasty below the penis. My wife says that the meta is the "workhorse." But now I have a "show horse" too.
>
> — *Trans man in his 60s*

Phallus Tattoos: A Game Changer

Tattoo art can provide a postphalloplasty appearance that better approximates the neighboring skin tone. Subtle color variegations bring the appearance of texture, and nearly hidden blue veins bring greater detail than ever possible. Shane Wallin of Garnet Tattoo in San Diego is one of a number of artists who does decorative tattooing, 3D nipple areolar pigmentation, and phallus tattoo art.

These photos show pre- and posttattoo results in an individual who had free flap phalloplasty by Jens Berli, MD, of Oregon Health and Science University Hospital in Portland, Oregon.

For more information on Wallin's services, search **garnettattoo.com**, or **ftmtattoo.com/phalloplasty**. Check with your surgeon as to when it is safe to tattoo after phalloplasty.

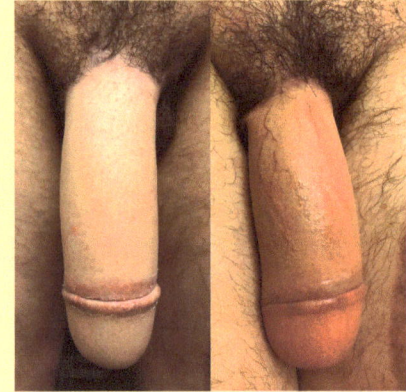

Figure 6.3. A phallus tattoo.

Quest House: A Post-Op Home for Transmasculine and Nonbinary Individuals Recovering from Phalloplasty and Other Gender-Affirming Surgeries near San Francisco

Meiko Xavier is the manager of Quest House in Pacifica, California. He writes an informative blog at myphalloplasty.wordpress.com, and he answered my questions about Quest House here on these next few pages. This email interview was conducted in October 2019. Learn more about Quest House at questhouseservices.wordpress.com.

> After this interview was completed, Quest House closed in May 2020 as a result of lease and COVID-19 complications. Meiko and I decided to leave this information in the book, partly because it beautifully describes the functions of a postsurgery recovery house and partly because it emphasizes the importance of such services.
>
> Then, as I was making my final review in July 2021, I learned that Quest House had reopened on a limited scale with expansion plans for the future. Check their website for information on their current situation: questhouseservices.wordpress.com. Hopefully, Quest House will have expanded capacity in the future and they will need our donations.
>
> — Linda Gromko, MD

Linda: I understand you just moved your location.

Meiko: Yes! We have been in our new location in Pacifica since May 1, 2019. We moved from a two-bedroom apartment in Sausalito to a five-bedroom, three-and-a-half-bathroom home.

Linda: Who stays at Quest House?

Meiko: About 70 percent of our guests are having Stage 1 phalloplasty, which is the construction of the phallus. (This varies from surgeon to surgeon.) For most, a Stage 1 phalloplasty is the biggest and most intense of the surgeries. Our guests usually stay for about 1 month and have a caregiver for at least 2 weeks. The other 30 percent are returning for future surgery stages or repairs or are having metoidioplasty. But all our guests are having gender-affirming lower surgeries.

Linda: What are your room rates?

Meiko: Our sliding scale is $75 to $125 per night. It is a self-selected sliding scale and we do not require any proof of income. We ask that people pay what they feel they are able to. We're hoping to be able to reduce the lower end of our sliding scale in the future. In the meantime, we're aiming to create an official scholarship fund sometime this year that we'd like to continue to grow.

Linda: How do you book rooms, and how many people can stay at one time?

Meiko: We book online, first-come, first-serve. We have four guest rooms, each with two beds, plus another room for our house host, who is always managing, supporting, and living in the space. We also have a sofa sleeper and a cot. We try not to overload the house since that makes navigating the bathrooms more challenging. We have three full bathrooms and one half-bath. The half-bath will be getting a shower added to it soon.

Linda: Do most guests have caregivers with them?

Meiko: People who are here for the microsurgery portion of phalloplasty need to plan to have someone care for them for a minimum of their first 2 weeks out of the hospital. This is a firm policy that our house has developed after trying a variety of ways of working with and supporting our guests.

In order to keep the house safe, each person having that big surgery just has to have someone there whose main priority is to help with their needs one-on-one. While not everyone needs around-the-clock support for the 2 full weeks (some need more and some need less), the average person ends up being very grateful that they had a dedicated support person during this time.

Each one of our bedrooms has two beds, and the caregiver stays in the same room. It's not unusual to have mothers come and support their sons. In fact, two of our four surgical guests staying with us right now are here with their mothers!

If a guest is not able to identify someone to help them during their recovery, we refer folks to a project with are in collaboration with called T4T (t4tcaregiving.org).

Linda: Are the T4T caregivers or other hired caregivers medical or nursing folks?

Meiko: T4T has caregivers who have been working as caregivers for many, many years—some for well over a decade. While they have some medical training, they are not nurses or CNAs (certified nurse assistants). There's a lot of transparency about this.

Linda: What trans health or medical training do they have?

Meiko: Oliver, the fellow that manages T4T, has more than 16 years of direct caregiving experience, ranging from adults and children with special needs and adults with dementia to end-of-life, HIV, and cancer care patients. He has 9 cumulative years of providing care for trans folks who are undergoing a range of gender-affirming procedures.

Linda: What is T4T's rate?

Meiko: $150 per day if someone wants an around-the-clock advocate during their hospital stay and $100 per day thereafter.

Linda: Is a staff person at Quest House all the time?

Meiko: Most of the time. Our host (which is usually me) spends probably 2 to 4 hours per day cleaning and turning over bedrooms for next guests, emailing with upcoming guests and helping them to prepare for their stay and surgery, and about 3 to 4 hours per day supporting the guests in the house and helping or teaching the caregivers how to support their people.

The host often takes guests to medical appointments and to the ER when emergencies arise. We also spend a fair amount of time providing emotional support; this is actually the largest task of the house host. (A guest's personal and medical needs are generally taken care of by their caregiver.)

Linda: Are caregivers able to administer antibiotics or provide more advanced home care?

Meiko: As someone who has worked in the mental health field in residential settings, I know that there is a subtle but important distinction between "administering a medication" and "assisting someone with their medications." We are definitely not "administering" medications at Quest House. We are simply providing the support that any family member, friend, or partner of a person having surgery would be doing for their loved one. We do suggest that people document their medications by using a medication log and writing down the times they last took a medication to reduce the likelihood of forgetting a med or taking one too frequently.

Linda: What medical supplies do people need to bring?

Meiko: There is a list on our website under the "Your Stay" tab. One of the benefits of our community space is that we have a lot of unopened supplies that end up being donated by previous guests. There is also a supplies list I created for my blog, *My Phalloplasty*, at myphalloplasty.wordpress.com/2016/09/28/medical-supplies-packing-list.

Linda: What kind of food is available?

Meiko: People prefer to purchase their own food for the most part. But sometimes folks will use Instacart to order groceries if they don't have a rental car. Uber Eats is a popular choice as well. There is also a fair amount of free food that gets donated when people check out.

Linda: How do you screen your guests?

Meiko: We screen 100 percent of our guests over the phone to make sure that we are a good fit for their needs and that we can meet their expectations. Quest House is a very intentional space. We are creating, protecting, and fostering a sacred healing environment. We hope to be accessible to a wide spectrum of folks who are arriving at this surgical process having gone through a variety of different life experiences or access to resources. We ultimately make decisions by relying on a deep sense of intuition and past experience with what has and hasn't worked for the house.

Linda: Are you supported at all by the surgeons whose patients you see?

Meiko: We have received donations from three different surgical teams as we were fundraising and getting ready to move. We'd love to secure sustaining donations for the future of this project from the surgical teams whose patients we continuously serve.

Linda: And does insurance cover Quest House for your guests?

Meiko: As far as insurance goes, we are not able to bill insurance companies directly since we are a community space and not a medical facility. However, many insurance companies (sometimes easily and sometimes with a lot of pressure) will reimburse folks for travel and lodging costs associated with accessing care when the circumstances require traveling a long distance from their home. The tricky thing is that most insurance companies have this benefit listed as specifically for "transplant patients." The irony is that phalloplasty patients technically are having a transplant surgery of sorts. Maybe in time, supportive community healing spaces like Quest House will be covered by insurance.

Linda: It sounds like guests have great experiences at Quest House.

Meiko: A little more than half of our guests return for one or more stays with us and about 25 percent return two or more times. The bonds formed here are strong. I like to call Quest House "the sweetest home you never had." For many (but not all of us), that's the truth. We take care of one another here. Many of our folks report never having experienced true community until staying with us.

I greatly appreciate Meiko Xavier's information. If you are able to support Quest House, donate through their website at questhouse.services/donate.

— Linda Gromko, MD

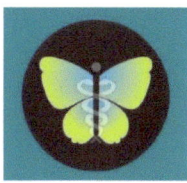

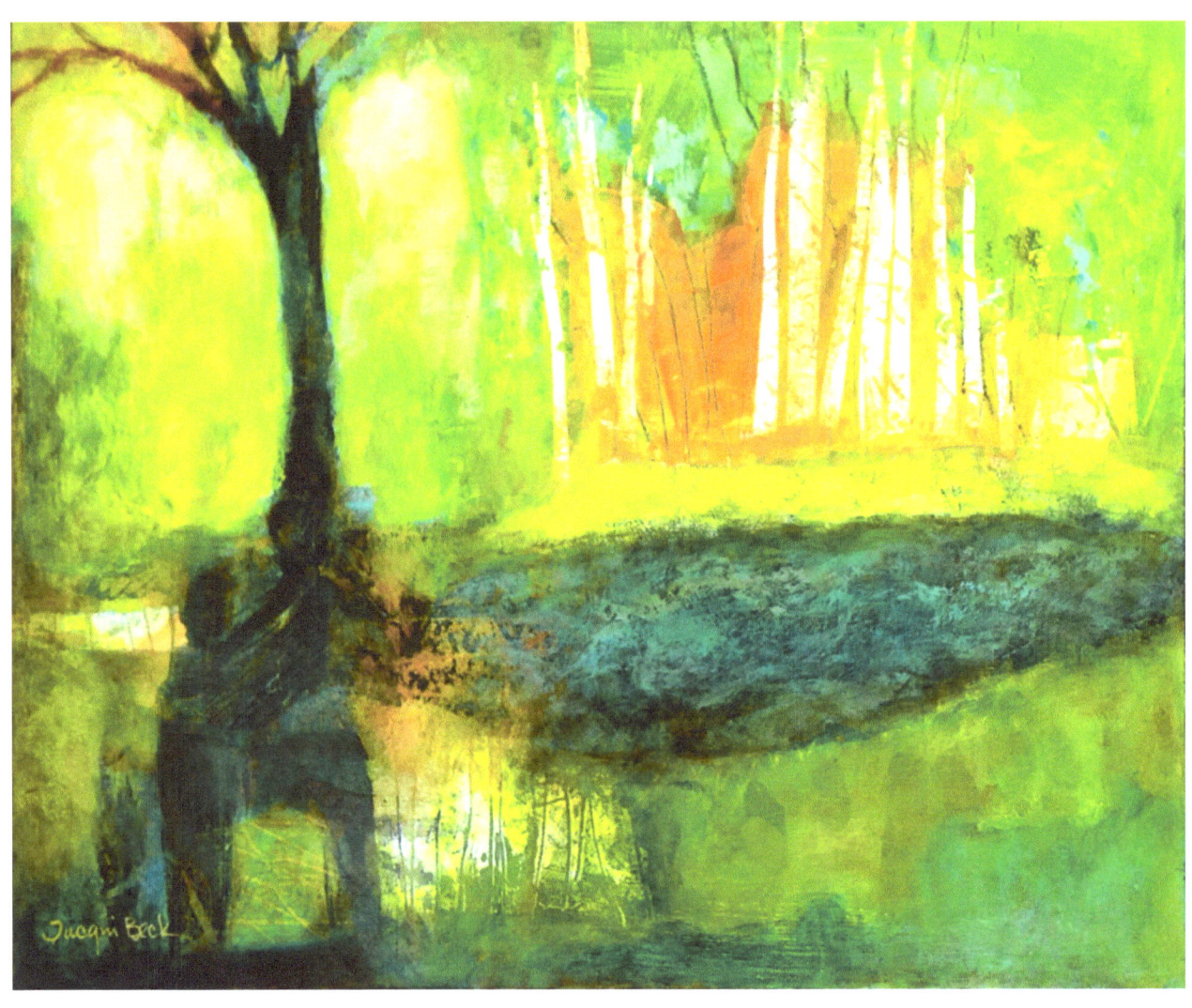

Still Forest

CONCLUSION

Gender-affirming surgery is an enormous step in an individual's life—easily the equivalent of a marriage, a graduation, or the birth of a child. Maybe someday, society will celebrate gender-affirming surgeries with parties and flowers, greeting cards, and how-to books to guide an individual through the experience. For now, information and education are important starting points.

As you come to the end of this important body of information, I sincerely hope it helps you as you make your own decisions about gender-affirming surgeries and as you recover from the surgeries themselves. If you have been reading in the interest of a partner, friend, or child, I hope this book makes you a stronger, better-informed advocate. And if you are a healthcare provider in any capacity, I hope this gives you the information you should have learned in professional school—but likely, never did.

Thank you for your time and consideration, and my very best wishes in your journey ahead.

— Linda Gromko, MD
   September 2022
   Seattle, Washington

LIST OF FIGURES AND TABLES

List of Figures

Figure 2.1	Stereotypically male and female faces.
Figure 2.2	Differences in the skulls of assigned males and females.
Figure 2.3	Facial feminization surgery.
Figure 2.4	Breast implants over and under the pectoralis muscle.
Figure 2.5	Embryologic equivalents in male and female external genitals.
Figure 2.6	Vaginoplasty 1 of 4.
Figure 2.7	Vaginoplasty 2 of 4.
Figure 2.8	Vaginoplasty 3 of 4.
Figure 2.9	Vaginoplasty 4 of 4.
Figure 2.10	The perineum in an AFAB and an AMAB.
Figure 2.11	The peritoneum in an AFAB and an AMAB.
Figure 2.12	Anatomy of the colon.
Figure 3.1	Tracheal augmentation.
Figure 3.2	Top-surgery scars.
Figure 3.3	Internal female reproductive organs.
Figure 3.4	Structure of the skin.
Figure 3.5	Forearm flap phalloplasty, Stage 1.
Figure 3.6	Forearm flap phalloplasty, Stage 2.
Figure 3.7	Forearm flap phalloplasty, Stage 3.
Figure 3.8	Delayed pedicle flap phalloplasty.
Figure 3.9	The penis/phallus-preserving vaginoplasty with peritoneal pull-through.
Figure 5.1	Resting on your side with extra pillow support.
Figure 5.2	Elevation of the legs.
Figure 6.1	*The Great Wall of Vagina* by Jamie McCartney.
Figure 6.2	A 3D nipple tattoo.
Figure 6.3	A phallus tattoo.

List of Tables

Table 3.1	Deciding on a type of male genital surgery.
Table 5.1	Protein content of various foods from animal and plant sources.

BIBLIOGRAPHY

Bertoluci, Marcello Casaccia, and Viviane Zorzanelli Rocha. "Cardiovascular Risk Assessment in Patients with Diabetes." *Diabetology & Metabolic Syndrome* 9, no. 25 (April 20, 2017), https://doi.org/10.1186/s13098-017-0225-1.

Bizic, Marta, Vladimir Kojovic, Dragana Duisin, Dusan Stanojevic, Svetlana Vujovic, Aleksandar Milosevic, Gradimir Korac, and Miroslav L. Djordjevic. "An Overview of Neovaginal Reconstruction Options in Male to Female Transsexuals." *The Scientific World Journal* 2014, Article ID 638919 (May 26, 2014): 8 pages. https://doi.org/10.1155/2014/638919.

Caceres, Vanessa. "9 Best Ways to Quit Smoking." *US News & World Report*. Last reviewed February 12, 2021. https://health.usnews.com/wellness/articles/best-ways-to-quit-smoking.

Capitán, Luis. "Management of Complex Revision Frontal Sinus and Forehead Cases." Lecture presented at the WPATH 26th Scientific Symposium Surgeon's Program, November 6, 2020.

Capitán, Luis, Javier Gutiérrez Santamaría, Daniel Simon, Devin Coon, Carlos Bailón, Raúl J. Bellinga, Thiago Tenório, and Fermín Capitán-Cañadas. "Facial Gender Confirmation Surgery: A Protocol for Diagnosis, Surgical Planning, and Postoperative Management." *Plastic and Reconstructive Surgery* 145, no. 4 (April 2020): 818e–28e. https://doi.org/10.1097/prs.0000000000006686.

De Luca, Maurizio, Luigi Angrisani, Jacques Himpens, Luca Busetto, Nicola Scopinaro, Rudolf Weiner, Alberto Sartori et al. "Indications for Surgery for Obesity and Weight-Related Diseases: Position Statements from the International Federation for the Surgery of Obesity and Metabolic Disorders (IFSO)." *Obesity Surgery* 26, no. 8 (July 2016): 1659–96. https://doi.org/10.1007/s11695-016-2271-4.

Deschamps-Braly, Jordan C., Caitlin L. Sacher, Jennifer Fick, and Douglas K. Ousterhout. "First Female-to-Male Facial Confirmation Surgery with Description of a New Procedure for Masculinization of the Thyroid Cartilage (Adam's Apple)." *Plastic & Reconstructive Surgery* 139, no. 4 (April 2017): 883e–87e. https://doi.org/10.1097/prs.0000000000003185.

Dowden, Richard V. "Transumbilical Breast Augmentation Is Safe and Effective." *Seminars in Plastic Surgery* 22, no. 1 (February 2008): 51–9. https://doi.org/10.1055/s-2007-1019143.

FSA Store. "Transgender Counseling or Surgery: FSA Eligibility." Accessed July 28, 2021. https://fsastore.com/FSA-Eligibility-List/T/Transgender-Counseling-or-Surgery-E717.aspx.

Games, Finlay. "Phalloplasty Final Stage | AMS Implant Review." *Finn the InFinncible*, May 25, 2019. http://finlaygames.com/phalloplasty-final-stage-ams-implant-review.

Gillis, Chelsia, and Paul E. Wischmeyer. "Preoperative Nutrition and the Elective Surgical Patient: Why, How and What?" *Anaesthesia* 74, Supplement 1 (January 2019): 27–35. https://doi.org/10.1111/anae.14506.

Grant, Jaime M., Lisa A. Mottet, and Justin Tanis. *National Transgender Discrimination Survey Report on Health and Health Care*. Washington DC: National Center for Transgender Equality, 2010. https://cancer-network.org/wp-content/uploads/2017/02/National_Transgender_Discrimination_Survey_Report_on_health_and_health_care.pdf.

Huang, Catherine K., and Neal Handel. "Effects of Singulair (Montelukast) Treatment for Capsular Contracture." *Aesthetic Surgery Journal* 30, no. 3 (July 2010): 404–8. https://doi.org/10.1177/1090820x10374724.

James, Sandy E., Jody L. Herman, Susan Rankin, Mara Keisling, Lisa Mottet, and Ma'ayan Anafi. *The Report of the 2015 U.S. Transgender Survey*. Washington, DC: National Center for Transgender Equality, 2016. https://transequality.org/sites/default/files/docs/usts/USTS-Full-Report-Dec17.pdf.

Kanhai, Robert C. J. "Sensate Vagina Pedicled-Spot for Male-to-Female Transsexuals: The Experience in the First 50 Patients." *Aesthetic Plastic Surgery* 40, no. 2 (February 18, 2016): 284–7. https://doi.org/10.1007/s00266-016-0620-2.

Kenney, William Larry, and Percy Chiu. "Influence of Age on Thirst and Fluid Intake." *Medicine and Science in Sports and Exercise* 33, no. 9 (October 2001): 1524–32. https://doi.org/10.1097/00005768-200109000-00016.

Kornfield, Meryl. "VA Plans to Offer Gender-Confirmation Surgery to Transgender Veterans, Reversing Ban." *The Washington Post*, June 19, 2021. https://www.washingtonpost.com/national-security/2021/06/19/veterans-gender-affirmation-surgery/.

Morche, Johannes, Tim Mathes, and Dawid Pieper. "Relationship Between Surgeon Volume and Outcomes: A Systematic Review of Systematic Reviews." *Systematic Reviews* 5, no. 1 (November 2016): 1–15. https://doi.org/10.1186/s13643-016-0376-4.

Nolan, Ian T., Christopher J. Kuhner, and Geolani W. Dy. "Demographic and Temporal Trends in Transgender Identities and Gender Confirming Surgery." *Translational Andrology and Urology* 8, no. 3 (June 2019): 184–90. doi: 10.21037/tau.2019.04.09.

Petrucelli, Nancie, Mary B. Daly, and Tuya Pal. "BRCA1- and BRCA2-Associated Hereditary Breast and Ovarian Cancer." In *GeneReviews*, edited by Margaret P. Adam et al. Seattle: University of Washington, 1993–2020, September 4, 1998, updated December 15, 2016. https://www.ncbi.nlm.nih.gov/books/NBK1247/.

Rodriguez, Alvaro H. "Male-to-Female Gender Affirming Surgery Using Nile Tilapia Fish Skin as a Biocompatible Graft." Presentation at the WPATH 26th Scientific Symposium Surgeon's Program, November 7, 2020.

Shaeer, Osama Kamal Zaki. "Shaeer's Technique: A Minimally Invasive Procedure for Monsplasty and Revealing the Concealed Penis," *PRS Global Open* 4, no. 8 (August 29, 2016): e1019. https://dx.doi.org/10.1097%2FGOX.0000000000001019.

Toomey, Russell B., Amy K. Syvertsen, and Maura Shramko. "Transgender Adolescent Suicide Behavior." *Pediatrics* 142, no. 4 (October 1, 2018): 2017–4218. https://doi.org/10.1542/peds.2017-4218.

Transgender Legal Defense and Education Fund. *Medical Necessity of Facial Gender Reassignment Surgery for Transgender Women: Literature Review*. Washington, DC: Transgender Legal Defense and Education Fund, September 10, 2020. https://transhealthproject.org/documents/34/Facial_surgery_medical_necessity_literature_review.pdf.

Under Armour. *Myfitnesspal*. V. 20.7.0.29453. 2020.

US Food and Drug Administration. "Risks and Complications of Breast Implants." Updated September 28, 2020. https://www.fda.gov/medical-devices/breast-implants/risks-and-complications-breast-implants#Capsular_Contracture.

PHOTO AND ILLUSTRATION CREDITS

Cover
Inattention to Detail, Jacqui Beck

Title Page
Holding the World, Jacqui Beck

Preface
Tree House, Jacqui Beck

Introduction
In the Trees, Jacqui Beck

Chapter 1 | Planning for Your Surgery
Many Socks, Jacqui Beck
Break Down Cigarette, Adobe Stock, Nopphon

Chapter 2 | Feminizing Surgeries
Conversation, Jacqui Beck
Business Is Good! [stereotypically male and female faces], iStock, Yuri_Arcurs
Male and Female Skulls, used with permission from Addicus Books; Douglas K. Ousterhout, Facial Feminization Surgery; A Guide for the Transgendered Woman, Omaha: Addicus Books, 2010
Facial Feminization Surgery, Hillary Wilson, hwilsonillustration.com
Breast Implant Over and Under, Bob Bost
Homologues of External Genitalia, Frank Netter, MD, Netterimages.com
Male-to-Female Vaginoplasty [four illustrations], Hillary Wilson, hwilsonillustration.com
Perineum Anatomy Engraving 1886, iStock, THEPALMER
Scheme of the Course of the Peritoneum in Women, iStock, ilbusca
Peritoneum (Male), iStock, ilbusca
Large Intestine, Colon Sections Labeled in Male Abdominal Anatomy, iStock, Hank Grebe

Chapter 3 | Masculinizing Surgeries
Birdhouse, Jacqui Beck
Tracheal Augmentation, Chris Gralapp, chrisgralapp.com
Top-Surgery Scars, Bob Bost
Female Reproductive System, iStock, 7activestudio
Structure of the Skin, iStock, Paladjai
Forearm Flap Phalloplasty [three illustrations], Hillary Wilson, hwilsonillustration.com
Pedicle Flap Phalloplasty Steps, Bob Bost
Penis-Preserving Peritoneal Pull-Through Vaginoplasty, Bob Bost

Chapter 4 | In Case of Emergencies
Inattention to Detail, Jacqui Beck

Chapter 5 | Taking Care of Yourself after Surgery
Comfort Found, Jacqui Beck
Resting on Your Side with Pillows, Bob Bost
Elevation of the Legs, Bob Bost

Chapter 6 | Specific Postoperative Circumstances Dealing with Specific Surgeries
Feels Like Home, Jacqui Beck
The Great Wall of Vagina, Panel 4, Jamie McCartney, jamiemccartney.com
Tyrannosaurus rex, iStock, Warpaintcobra
Pink Pockets, courtesy of Pink Pockets, pink-pockets.com
3D nipple tattoo, courtesy of the Vinnie Myers Team, vinniemyersteam.com
Saline Solution, iStock, kckate16
Phalloplasty tattoos, courtesy of FTM Tattoo, ftmtattoo.com/phalloplasty

Conclusion
Still Forest, Jacqui Beck

About the Author
Linda Gromko portrait, Erica Sciarretta, Sorella Photos, sorellaphotos.com
Jacqui Beck portrait, Akasha Schutz

ACKNOWLEDGMENTS

Gender-Affirming Surgeries: Planning through Post-op for Transgender and Gender-Nonconfirming Adults was modified in September 2022 from *A Practical Reference for Transgender and Gender-Nonconforming Adults*. It was felt that a more focused and more compact book would better serve the individual seeking support before and after gender-affirming surgery. The "big book" simply grew out of control—and serves as a casual but comprehensive text on transgender health.

Both of these books have brought together a committed group of professionals and an email reunion of the folks who contributed their talents to create *Where's MY Book? A Guide for Transgender and Gender Non-Conforming Youth, Their Parents, & Everyone Else.*

I acknowledge the copy and design editing completed by author and editor Mi Ae Lipe. Mi Ae also executed the important task of fact-checking and elevated the graphic design and subject matter integration to a level I'd only envisioned. This book combined the best medical illustrations I could find, plus photographs, graphs, complex medical content, and a hodgepodge of personal stories—beautifully drawn together by Mi Ae into a credible whole. I am further grateful for Mi Ae's gentle midwifery in the enormous tasks of locating the proper ebook integrator and printers who made all the difference in getting this book out to the world. Thank you for your patience, Mi Ae.

I am grateful to my long-time friend Bob Bost. Bob's line drawings offer more medical clarity, helping me to explain tough concepts more effectively. Our butterfly logo, also Bob's design, is the registered trademark representing our practice. Combining the medical caduceus and the butterfly for transformation, Bob captured the essence of what we do.

Jacqui Beck's art is represented on the cover and sprinkled through this book, giving it more dimension and passion. What a joy to have her paintings in a book yet again. Read more about Jacqui's work on page 157. Thanks also to Richard Nicol, who photographed these paintings.

I recognize all my coworkers at Queen Anne Medical Associates and Transformative Aesthetics for weathering another book project. Most especially, I recognize and thank office manager Barbara Boni and Suzi Spinner, the director of Queen Anne Medical Electrolysis and Laser. Thanks to Carol Keenholts, ARNP, our outstanding nurse practitioner—and to all of our staff.

I am grateful to Marsha Botzer, the founder of Seattle's internationally known Ingersoll Gender Center, for her mentorship, her foreword for the "big book," and a friendship that spans decades.

I extend grateful thanks to my longtime friend and cadaver partner Andrew M. Faulk, MD for his considerable personal and financial support.

As in the first book, I called on a village of professionals in trans medicine and related fields. These folks took their time to review my chapters and make additions and corrections. One of the surgeons, when asked to review this work, said, "It's a pandemic. I have some time on my hands!" These folks made their contributions with no expectation of remuneration—it was simply to add to the collective knowledge and to serve people, and they are listed here. And there must be people who have been inadvertently omitted; I thank them and ask their forgiveness.

I am supremely grateful to the following professionals who served as volunteer consultants and contributors for this book. In most cases, they reviewed specific chapters dealing with areas of expertise for accuracy. They often added comments, which are generally noted as quotations in the text. They are listed here in the approximate order of their appearance in the book. Contact and credential information may be found on their respective websites. Certain individuals are listed for other informational contributions.

Marsha Botzer	ingersollgendercenter.org
Aidan Key	genderdiversity.org
E. Antonio Mangubat, MD	labelleviecosmetic.com
Toby R. Meltzer, MD	themeltzerclinic.com
Ryan Tennant, DDS	2thstudio.com
Robert Niedbalski, DO	hairreplacementsurgeon.com
Richard Santucci, MD	cranects.com
Curtis Crane, MD	cranects.com
Noah E. Lewis, Esq.	linkedin.com/in/noahelewis
Christine McGinn, DO	drchristinemcginn.com
M. Dru Lavasseur, Esq.	linkedin.com/in/mdlevasseur
Marci L. Bowers, MD	marcibowers.com
Jordan Deschamps-Braly, MD	deschamps-braly.com
Fermín Capitán, PhD	facialteam.eu
Scott Mosser, MD	genderconfirmation.com
Douglas K. Ousterhout, MD	deschamps-braly.com/dr-ousterhout-facial-feminization-surgeon-ffs
Thomas Satterwhite, MD	alignsurgical.com
Heidi Wittenberg, MD	mozaiccare.net
Geoffrey Stiller, MD	stilleraesthetics.com
Alvaro H. Rodriguez, MD	cecmcolombia.com
Harlowe Rayne Thunderword-Cohen	linkedin.com/in/harlowerayne-thunderword-cohen-4aba0b11a
Dev Gurjala, MD	alignsurgical.com
Finlay Games	finlaygames.com
Jamie McCartney	jamiemccartney.com
Vinnie Myers	vinniemyersteam.com
Shane Wallin	garnettattoo.com
Meiko Xavier	questhouseservices.wordpress.com
Ellie Zara Ley, MD	themeltzerclinic.com

Gratitude to Our Financial Contributors

Finally, many thanks to the individuals who donated to my GoFundMe campaign—guardian angels do exist! While I did not include names of individuals out of respect for privacy, I must recognize Dr. Bob Niedbalski, Dr. Andrew Faulk, and David Hamilton for their extraordinary contributions!

While some of the surgeons contributed to the GoFundMe campaign, I singled none of them out, as I didn't want to infer that their inclusion was "encouraged." Nonetheless, contributions are still welcome to support the extensive costs of writing and printing books like these.

I invite anyone wishing to contribute to cover book printing expenses and promotion to go to GoFundMe.com and search "Linda Gromko transgender book." (And thank you.)

INDEX

Page numbers with an *f* refer to a figure or a caption; *t* refers to a table; and *n* indicates a footnote.

A

acetaminophen 105
Adam's apple
    enhancement of 65
    Facialteam protocol for 34
    implant for 63
    male/female differences in 31
    and tracheal shave 33
adolescents, parental consent for 19
alcohol consumption 11
Allen Carr's Easy Way to Quit Smoking Without Willpower 9
allergic reaction (anaphylaxis) 91, 92
AMAB (assigned male at birth). *See* assigned male at birth
anaplastic large-cell lymphoma 41
anastomoses, stricture/fistula risk of 74, 82
aorta, location of 56
aseptic, definition of 111
aspirin
    for pain 105
    presurgical cessation of 21
assigned female at birth (AFAB)
    genitals identified at birth 47f
assigned male at birth (AMAB)
    and genitals identified at birth 47f
augmentation mammoplasty. *See* breast enlargement

B

baldness 31
bariatric surgery
    skin removal after 42
    for weight loss 11
BBL (Brazilian butt lift). *See* Brazilian butt lift
Berli, Jens 134
BIA-ALCL (breast implant-associated anaplastic large-cell lymphoma) 41
BII (breast implant illness) 40
bilateral salpingo-oophorectomy
    overview 69–70
    metoidioplasty with 75
    with phalloplasty 130
    procedures for 127–28
binders. *See* chest binders
bleeding, as emergency 92
blepharoplasty, Facialteam protocol for 34
blood clot risks
    reduction of
        with compression devices 131
    sources of
        estradiol 22
        surgery 6
BMI (body mass index) 10–11
body contouring
    lifting and filling 43–44
    nonsurgical 41
    risks of 42
    surgical 41–42
body mass index (BMI) 10–11
bone age test 34
Bosted, Christopher xv
Botzer, Marsha xiv
Bowers, Marci 3, 15, 22
Brazilian butt lift (BBL)
    mortality from 44
    process 43
BRCA1/BRCA2 mutations 68, 69, 127
breast cancer
    screening for 68, 128
breast enlargement
    with estrogen 36
    with implants. *See* breast implants
    postsurgical care 119
    with progesterone 36
breast implant illness (BII) 40
breast implant-associated anaplastic large-cell lymphoma (BIA-ALCL) 41
breast implants
    choices/sizing 36–37, 38–39
    complications/risks of 39–41
    saline/silicone 37
    surgery 37–38
breast modification, presurgery letters 19
breathing problems/asthma 91–92, 118
brow bones
    enhancing 65
    male/female differences in 31, 63
    surgical changes to 33
brows
    male/female differences in 31
    surgical changes to 33
bupropion (Wellbutrin) 8, 9
Burou, Georges 49
butt-contouring implants 44

C

Capitán, Luis 34
capsular contracture grading scale (Baker scale) 39–40
cardiology exam 5
    See also heart disease
Caring Bridge 102
carry letters 23
cervix
    removal of 69, 79, 127
Chantix (varenicline) 8–9
cheekbones
    implants 33, 65
    male/female differences in 31

chest binders
    after surgery 126
chest pain 93
chest reconstruction (top surgery)
    overview 66–68
    postsurgical 126–27
    types of
        double incision surgery 66–68
        keyhole surgery 67
children
    gender asynchrony awareness xvi
    transgender xv
chin
    contouring 33
    implants in 34
    male/female differences in 31
    surgical changes to 33
Christophersen, Lauren xvii
climax. *See* orgasm
clitoris
    defined hood over 53
    embryologic 47f
    glans penis as male equivalent 46, 72
    metoidioplasty changes to 74
codeine 104
colon, anatomy of 58f
colonoscopies, after right-colon vaginoplasty 59
compression
    devices 131
    garments 42, 118
    stockings 26
constipation 109
CoolSculpting 41
cost
    of gender-affirming surgeries. *See* gender-affirming surgeries
    See also insurance coverage
coumadin (Warfarin) 6
counseling
    provider lists. *See* Ingersoll Gender Center
COVID-19 test requirements 98
Crane Center, surgery volume and experience 18
cricothyroid approximation 34, 36
cross-sex hormones
    before vaginoplasty 54
    in young adolescents xvi
cryolipolysis. *See* CoolSculpting

D

Davydov, S. N. 55
deep vein thromboses (DVTs)
    as surgical risk 6
dehydration 108
Deschamps-Braly, Jordan 23, 63, 65
Deutsch, Madeline 22
dilation
    after surgery 120–23
    lubrication during 52
Dilaudid (hydromorphone) 104

direct oral anticoagulants (DOACs) 6
disabled parking permits 25
DOACs (direct oral anticoagulants) 6
Dowden, Richard V. 38
drains. *See* postsurgical drains
DVTs (deep vein thromboses). *See* deep vein thromboses

E

electrolysis
    equipment for xvii
    in-house xvii
    pain management xvii–xviii
endoscopic glottoplasty (Wendler glottoplasty) 36
endoscopic vocal cord shortening 34
endotracheal tube (ET tube) 36
estradiol
    presurgery 22
    prostate changes from 53
    See also ethinyl estradiol
estrogen
    breast enlargement with 36
ET tube (endotracheal tube) 36
ethinyl estradiol 22
eunuchs 89
eye swelling, postsurgical 117

F

facelift 34, 66
facial feminization surgery (FFS)
    overview 30–34, 35f
    imaging use in 32
    postsurgical care 117–19
    skulls of assigned males and females 32f
    stereotypical male and female faces 30f
facial masculinization surgery (FMS) 63–66
facial surgery
    hair removal preceding 23
    presurgery letters 20
Facialteam (Spain) 32, 34, 117, 118
fallopian tubes
    location of 56
    removal of 69, 79, 127
Family and Medical Leave Act (FMLA) paperwork 23–24
fat grafting 34
FDA adverse event reporting 40
female reproductive organs 69f
feminizing surgeries
    body contouring. *See* body contouring
    breast enlargement. *See* breast enlargement
    facial. *See* facial feminization surgery
    genital. *See* genital surgeries
Ferraiolo, Tony 15
fetal development
    male and female external genitals 47f
fever 94
FFS (facial feminization surgery). *See* facial feminization surgery
fistulas
    overview 75
    resolution of 74–75, 75

flaps 76–77
fluid needs 108–09
FMLA (Family and Medical Leave Act) paperwork 23–24
FMS (facial masculinization surgery) 63–66
forehead
    3D reconstruction of 32
    elongation 65
    Facialteam protocol for 34
    male/female differences in 31

G

gabapentin (Neurontin) 105–6
Games, Finlay 87
Garnet Tattoo 134
Gender Diversity xv
gender nullification surgery ("the Smoothie") 89
Gender Odyssey xv
gender-affirming surgeries
    overview
        benefits/risks of 3
        goals of 2, 3, 33, 72–3, 73t
        surgery sequencing 2–3
        See also feminizing surgeries; masculinizing surgeries
    cost of
        overview 12–16
        insurance coverage for. *See* insurance coverage
        military coverage 14
        other funding sources 12–16
        as tax-deductible 13n6
    infections after surgery 23, 133
    medical evaluation/preparation
        about 3
        cardiology screening 5
        coagulation problems 6
        EKG 23
        hair removal xvii, 11–12
        immunization status 12
        lab tests 4
        medical conditions assessment 4–5
        physical fitness 12
        screening tests 5
        STD resolution 11
        weight loss 9–11
    nonsurgical expenses
        living expenses 13
        travel expenses 13–14
    preoperative confirmations (6 weeks prior)
        logistical arrangements 20–21
        medical arrangements 21–23
        travel arrangements 23
        work arrangements 23–24
    presurgery letters 19–20
    shopping lists for 27
    smoking cessation 7–9
    surgeon qualifications & selection 16–19
genital surgeries
    feminizing
        orchiectomy 44–45, 119
        vaginoplasty. *See* vaginoplasty

    masculinizing
        overview 72–74, 73t
        metoidioplasty. *See* metoidioplasty
        phalloplasty. *See* phalloplasty
    nonbinary 88–89
    preliminaries
        hair removal 54
        presurgery letters 19
    recovery time 102
genitals
    embryologic 47f
    female 47f
    male 47f
glans penis
    clitoris as female equivalent 46, 72
    embryologic 47f
glansplasty
    as glans penis creation 80, 86
    timing of 81, 85
GoFundMe 15
grafts
    fat grafting 34
    in implants 63, 65
    in phalloplasty. *See* phalloplasty
    skin. *See* skin grafts
    in vaginoplasty. *See* vaginoplasty
The Great Wall of Vagina 120
Gurjala, Dev 87

H

hair transplants
    in facial feminization 33
    in facial masculinization 65
hairlines, male/female differences in 31, 63
Harry Benjamin Society. *See* WPATH
health insurance. *See* insurance coverage
heart disease
    cardiology exam for 5
heparin 6
histrelin, before vaginoplasty 54
hormones
    for feminization
        estradiol. *See* estradiol
        testosterone blockers. *See* spironolactone
    for masculinization. *See* testosterone
    presurgery 22
    progesterone. *See* progesterone
    puberty blockers. *See* puberty blockers
    spironolactone (Aldactone). *See* spironolactone
    therapist letter in support of xiv, xv
hypercoagulable state 6
hypnotherapy, for smoking cessation 9
hysterectomy
    overview 69–70
    with metoidioplasty 75
    with phalloplasty 130
    procedures for 127–28

I

ibuprofen 105
I'll Show You Mine (Robertson) 120
immunization status 12
implants
    breast. *See* breast implants
    for butt-contouring. *See* butt-contouring implants
    facial 65
    Facialteam protocol for 34
    graft from a patient's rib 63, 65
incontinence 70
infection indicators 112, 133
inferior vena cava, location of 56
Ingersoll Gender Center
    founding of xiv
    as self-help organization xiv
    surgeons listed with 16
    therapist list 20
injections
    Facialteam protocol for 34
    for increasing volume 44
insurance coverage
    for chest reconstruction (top surgery) 66, 126
    for facial surgery 20
    for gender-affirming surgeries 1
    for genital surgeries 72
    for liposuction 42
    of transitioning xv
    types of 12–13, 14
intubation, vocal cord damage from 36

J

Jackson-Pratt bulb 112, 127
jaws
    Facialteam protocol for 34
    male/female differences in 31, 63
Jim Collins Foundation 15

K

Key, Aidan xv–xvi
kidneys
    infections 123–24
    location of 56
Kybella injections 41

L

labia majora, scrotum as male equivalent 46
labia minora
    embryologic 47f
    perineal raphe (ridge) as male equivalent 46
    refining 53
labiaplasty 53
laparoscopy 55, 88
laryngoplasty 34, 36
LaserLipo 41
Lehman, Robert xvi
LeVasseur, Dru 15
Lewis, Noah 13
liposuction 41–42, 70

lips
    Facialteam protocol for 34
    implants in 34
    male/female differences in 31
    surgical changes to 33
Lotsa Helping Hands 26, 101
low-molecular-weight heparin (Lovanox) 6–7, 22
Lupron-Depot blockade, before vaginoplasty 54

M

male sexual reassignment surgery. *See* masculinizing surgeries
mandible
    contouring 33, 65
Mangubat, E. Antonio 15, 40
masculinizing surgeries
    chest reconstruction (top surgery). *See* chest reconstruction
    facial. *See* facial masculinization surgery
    genital. *See* genital surgeries
    hysterectomy. *See* hysterectomy
    salpingo-oophorectomy. *See* bilateral salpingo-oophorectomy
McCartney, Jamie 120
McGinn, Christine 14, 15
Meal Train 101
Mediterranean diet 10
Meltzer, Toby xviii, 7, 31, 67, 84
metoidioplasty
    overview 74
    expectations for 75–76
    postsurgical care 129
    risks of 129
    types of
        with Centurion technique 74
        ring 74
        scrotoplasty with/without testicular implants 75
        with urethral lengthening 74–75, 129–30
Metzger, Dan xv
Metzger, Julie xvi
monsplasty 70, 128
Mosser, Scott 38

N

naproxen 105
narcotic pain relievers 104–05
nausea/vomiting/diarrhea 94
Neurontin (gabapentin) 105–06
911 calls
    overview 91–93
    allergic reaction (anaphylaxis) 92
nipples and areolas
    in chest reconstruction (male) 66, 67
    tattoos 127, 127f
non-Hodgkin's lymphoma 41
Noom (weight loss) 10
noses
    Facialteam protocol for 34
    male/female differences in 31
    rhinoplasty 33, 34, 65

NSAIDs
    cessation of 21
    for pain 105
nutrition
    after facial feminization 117
    fluids 108–09
    by IV 131
    protein requirements 106–08, 107t
    in wound healing 110

O

opiates 104–06
orchiectomy
    postsurgical care 119
    surgery 44–45
orgasm
    after transitioning 46, 54
ovaries
    location of 56, 69f
    removal of 69, 79, 127

P

pain management
    benzocaine, lidocaine, tetracaine (BLT) xviii
    constipation resulting from 109, 124
    dental blocks xviii
    in home care
        acetaminophen 105
        after facial feminization 117
        gabapentin (Neurontin) 105–06
        ice packs 26, 117, 119, 124, 129
        narcotics/tramadol 104–05, 106
        NSAIDs 105
        opiates 104–05
        severity/changes in 93
    in hospital
        patient-controlled analgesia (PCA) 100, 131
        types of 100
    referred pain 128
    scrotal field blocks xviii
    spermatic cord blocks xviii
pectoralis muscle, breast implants under/over 37–38, 37f
penis
    removal of 89
Percocet (oxycodone + acetaminophen) 104
Percodan (oxycodone + aspirin) 104
perineal raphe (ridge), labia minora as female equivalent 46
perineum, peritoneum vs. 55
peritoneum
    in AFAB 56–57, 56f
    in AMAB 56f
    definition of 55
    perineum vs. 55
PEs (pulmonary emboli). See pulmonary emboli
phalloplasty
    complications/risks of 87
    flaps
        delayed pedicle 77, 78
        free 77, 78
        pedicle 77, 78

grafts
    overview 76
    donor site 77
    full-thickness/split-thickness 77
    hair removal preceding xvii, 79, 84
    infection indicators 133
    postsurgical care 130–33
    removal of uterus, fallopian tubes, ovaries 127
    skin structure 78f
    types of
        anterior lateral thigh (ALT) flap 78, 84, 130–33
        delayed pedicle flap 78, 84–86, 85f, 133
        radial forearm flap (RFF). See radial forearm flap
photos of family members 32
physical fitness 12
Point of Pride 15, 127
postsurgical drains
    Jackson-Pratt bulb 112, 127
    removing 128
progesterone
    breast development with 36
prostate
    after transitioning 53
puberty
    female. See assigned female at birth
    male. See assigned male at birth
puberty blockers
    implantable histrelin xvi
    before vaginoplasty 54
pulmonary emboli (PEs)
    as surgical risk 6

Q

Quest House 101, 135–38
Quit Smoking programs. See smoking cessation

R

radial forearm flap (RFF)
    about 78
    stage 1: phallus creation 79–80, 80f
    stage 2: urethral lengthening and scrotoplasty 81, 81f
    stage 3: erectile implant 82, 83f
    postsurgical care 130–33
reduction mammoplasty 66
relationships, redefining xv
RFF (radial forearm flap). See radial forearm flap
rhinoplasty (nose job) 33, 65, 118
rice test for breast sizing 38–39
Robertson, Wrenna 120
robot-assisted surgery 70
Rodriguez, Alvaro H. 60

S

salpingo-oophorectomy, bilateral See bilateral salpingo-oophorectomy
Santucci, Richard 12, 18, 82, 84
Satterwhite, Thomas 40
scalp advance, hairline changes from 33
scrotal sac, reduction of 89
scrotal tissue, in vaginoplasty 45

scrotoplasty with prosthetic testes 130
scrotum
    embryologic 75f
    enlargement of 75
    labia majora as female equivalent 46
second opinions 2
sex and relationships
    post-op sex 122–23
sex hormones. *See* hormones
sexual intimacy, lubrication during 52
sexually transmitted diseases (STDs). *See* sexually transmitted infections
sexually transmitted infections (STIs) 11
SignUpGenius 101
silicone
    breast implants 37
    injection risks 44
Simon, Daniel 34
skin grafts
    microsurgical connection of 131
    in phalloplasty 76–77
    in vaginoplasty 88–89
smoking cessation 7–9, 34, 66–67, 126
speculum exams after surgery 122
STDs (sexually transmitted diseases). *See* STIs
sterile, definition of 111
Stiller, Geoffrey 58–59
STIs (sexually transmitted infections) 11
strictures, resolution of 74–75, 82
subglandular/subpectoral breast implants 37f
suicide
    ideation/thoughts of 93
    statistics xvi, xvin1
surgeon waiting lists 1
surgery
    hospital care
        admission/procedures 98
        postoperative 99–100
        in recovery 99
    infection indicators 112, 123–24, 133
    pain management. *See* pain management
    physical activity 118, 126
    postoperative home care
        overview 100–02
        care partner 132
        dressings/bandages 111–13
        fluid needs 108–09
        pet sleeping arrangements 103
        protein 107–08, 107t
        rest and relaxation 102–04, 103f
        sleep positions 103f, 126
        supplies for 103
        support system 101–02
        wound healing 110–13
        See also nutrition
    postoperative mental health care
        overview 113
        depression indicators 114
        911 calls 91–93
        suicidal thoughts 93
    risks
        from blood clots 6
        of breast cancer 6, 92
        from pulmonary embolism (blood clot in a lung) 6, 92
        other urgent situations 93–94
    sex after surgery 122–23
    specific surgeries
        bilateral salpingo-oophorectomy 69–70, 127–28, 130
        breast enlargement 119
        chest reconstruction (top surgery) 126–27
        facial feminization 117–19
        facial masculinization 126
        hysterectomy 127–28, 130
        metoidioplasty 129
        metoidioplasty with urethral lengthening 129–30
        monsplasty 128
        orchiectomy 119
        phalloplasty 130–33
        scrotoplasty with prosthetic testes 130
        vaginectomy 129
        vaginoplasty 119–25
    See also feminizing surgeries; masculinizing surgeries

T

tattoos
    nipples and areolas 67, 127, 127f
    phallus 134, 134f
T-cell lymphoma 41
temples, implants in 34
Tennant, Ryan xviii
testicles
    removal of 44–45, 89
testosterone
    early information on xv
    physical changes with
        Adam's apple prominence 31
        clitoral enlargement 72, 74
        facial changes as response to 30, 63
        vaginal bleeding, elimination 128
thromboembolism, unaltered 22
thrombophilias 6
Thunderword-Cohen, Harlowe Rayne 68
thyroid cartilage. *See* Adam's apple
tissue expanders
    after scrotoplasty 130
    in the scrotum 75, 82
To Quiet Inflammation (weight loss) 10
tracheal augmentation 64f
tracheal shave 33
Tramadol (Ultram) 106
transgender individuals
    children xiv
    "gatekeeping" xiv
Transgender Legal Defense and Education Fund 13, 20
TransHeartline House 101
transitioning
    insurance coverage of xv
    struggles of xv
tumescent liposuction 42
tummy tucks 42, 88–89

Tylenol 105

U
Ultram (Tramadol) 106
urinary symptoms 94
urinary tract/kidney infections 123–24
urination
    after metoidioplasty 129
    after vaginoplasty 123
    catheter for 129, 130, 132
    incontinence 70
uterus
    location of 56
    removal of 69, 79, 127

V
vaginal bleeding 128
vaginectomies
    about 79
    with metoidioplasty 75
    with phalloplasty 129
    postsurgical care 129
    timing of 81
    urethral lengthening risk reduction with 75
vaginoplasty
    overview 45–48
    constipation 124
    dilation after surgery 120–22
    grafts
        from lateral flank or abdominal areas 54, 55
        from tilapia 60
    granulation treated with silver nitrate 125
    hair removal preceding xvii, 11, 54, 59
    infections, urinary tract/kidney 123–24
    penis/phallus-preserving
        with full-thickness skin graft 88–89
        peritoneal pull-through 88, 88f
    postsurgical care 119–25
    risks of 55
    scrotal tissue use in 55
    speculum exams after surgery 122
    supplies for 187
    sutures coming out 125
    swelling in the perineum 124
    types of
        bowel 57n58
        intestinal 57n58
        with limited graft tissue 54
        limited-depth or zero-depth 54
        penile inversion 49–53, 49f
        penile inversion plus labiaplasty 215
        peritoneal pull-through 54, 55–57, 88, 88f
        rectosigmoid 57, 57n
        right-colon 58–59, 58f
    urination 123

vaginal bleeding 125
varenicline (Chantix) 8–9
vasoconstriction, and nicotine replacement products 8
Vicodin (hydrocodone + acetaminophen) 104
Vinnie Myers Team nipple tattoos 127
vitamin E cessation 21
vocal feminization surgery 34, 36
volume depletion 108
vulvoplasties 54

W
Wallin, Shane 134
Warfarin (coumadin) 6
weight loss 9–11
Weight Watchers 10
Wellbutrin (bupropion) 8, 9
Wendler glottoplasty (endoscopic glottoplasty) 36
Where's MY Book? A Guide for Transgender and Gender Non-Conforming Youth, Their Parents, & Everyone Else (Gromko) xvi, xvii, xxi
Will Puberty Last My Whole Life? (Metzger & Lehman) xvi–xvii
Wilson, Hillary 49, 79
Wittenberg, Heidi 55
World Professional Association for Transgender Health (WPATH). *See* WPATH
wound healing, foods for 25, 106–08
wound VAC (vacuum-assisted closure) 133
WPATH (World Professional Association for Transgender Health)
    as clearinghouse for clinicians xiv
    standards 45
    standards updating 19
    surgeons listed with 16
    therapist list 20

X
Xavier, Meiko 135–38

ABOUT THE AUTHOR

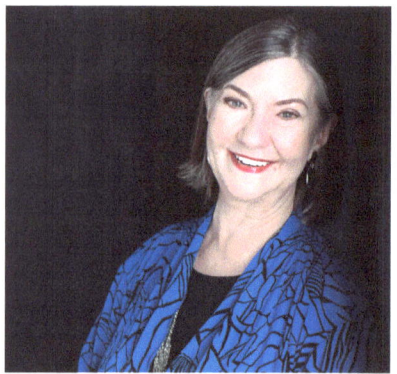

Linda Gromko, MD is a board-certified family practice physician who has worked with the transgender community since 1998, when a caller asked, "Does Dr. Gromko treat transgender women?" Dr. Gromko replied, "Not yet."

Thus began a decades-long commitment to transgender healthcare and education. Early experiences are discussed in the preface of this book, *Gender-Affirming Surgeries: Planning through Post-op for Transgender and Gender-Nonconforming Adults*. Today, she is one of the few Seattle physicians who treats transgender folk of all ages, along with the rest of her broad-ranging family practice.

Dr. Gromko's interest in healthcare goes back to the age of 14 when she volunteered as a candy striper. She earned both her bachelor's and master's degrees in nursing from the University of Washington. While working as a nurse practitioner at Planned Parenthood in Seattle, Dr. Gromko began her premed classes and enrolled in the University of Washington School of Medicine when her son Tim was only 4 years old.

After graduation from the University of Washington Family Medicine Residency program, Dr. Gromko worked in a large emergency room and a number of women's clinics while setting up her own practice, which opened in 1989. Initially, the practice focused on women's healthcare and obstetrics. Dr. Gromko stopped delivering babies in 2005.

In mid-life, Dr. Gromko found the love of her life in Steve Williams. When Steve's health plummeted as a result of diabetic kidney failure, Dr. Gromko quickly learned to perform home kidney dialysis, which the couple did for more than 3 years before Steve's death in 2011. The experience of providing home care to a critically ill spouse made Dr. Gromko a bit of a zealot in promoting home kidney dialysis, as well as in preventing diabetes and kidney failure. Her two memoirs about this period won several awards, as did the award-winning guide, *Arranging Your Life When Dialysis Comes Home: The Underwear Factor*, written with interior designer Jane C. McClure.

Dr. Gromko loves to speak about transgender health and welcomes speaking invitations.

She makes her home in Seattle and spends free time kayaking, riding a "bike that goes nowhere," and writing.

Linda@LindaGromkoMD.com
LindaGromkoMD.com (Website and blog)
QueenAnneMedicalAssociates.com (Office)

ABOUT ARTIST JACQUI BECK

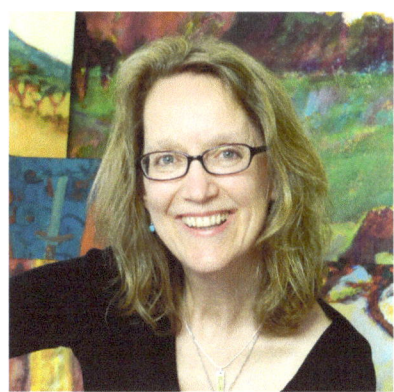

Jacqui Beck is an artist, art educator, and creativity coach living in Seattle, Washington. She has been teaching students of all ages for more than 15 years and is an adjunct professor of art at Seattle Pacific University. Her award-winning expressive acrylic paintings are collected and exhibited in the United States, Canada, Europe, and New Zealand. She has a master's degree in counseling psychology from the University of Victoria and is a trained life coach and creativity coach. She has studied at the Gage Academy of Art and with many nationally known artists.

In Jacqui Beck's words,

> "I create paintings using acrylics and mixed media. My artwork is colorful, personal, and expressive, and I keep in mind both the depth and whimsy of life. I often paint animal totem protectors representing the fierce strength of ourselves and those who love us. This strength, ideally, is tempered by a sense of paradox, irony, and humor. We can't always recognize our protectors by their appearance (notice chickens, birds, cats, and various strange or imaginary animals). The most powerful beings have an understanding of, and compassion for, our uniqueness and fallibility.
>
> "Like life, painting is an unfolding process of intention and accident. I notice what shows up and decide what to keep or enhance, and what to prune. The subject matter and meaning of my paintings are an exploration of what being a person means to me. I paint to explore my questions about life, about strength, fear, confusion, curiosity, and joy."

Jacqui Beck's project, Gender Personal, explores and celebrates gender variance through art, poetry, and recorded interviews. Its vision is to lead to social change and acceptance and to foster understanding by increasing awareness of the natural experience of gender variance. As the mother of a transgender son, Jacqui has a personal connection with this work. Many of the paintings in this book and in Gromko's earlier *Where's MY Book?* were done as part of the Gender Personal Project (genderpersonal.org). For more information on Jacqui Beck's more recent work, visit her website at jacquibeck.com.

www.ingramcontent.com/pod-product-compliance
Lightning Source LLC
Chambersburg PA
CBHW042346300426
44110CB00032B/43